PROGRAMMED INSTRUCTION HANDBOOK

NONDESTRUCTIVE TESTING

Ultrasonic

VOLUME III - APPLICATIONS

Published by **PH D**iversified, Inc.
5040 Highway 49 South
Harrisburg, NC 28075

Printed in the United States of America
ISBN 1-886630-06-2

ACKNOWLEDGMENTS

Publishing and Printing

Revision Editor: . . . . Dr. George Pherigo, *PH D*iversified, Inc.

Production Editor . . Ms. Mary Lou Hollifield, *PH D*iversified, Inc.

Proofreading . . . . Ms. Jean Pherigo, *PH D*iversified, Inc.
Proofreading . . . . Ms. Dana Smilie

Technical Content Revision

Technical Editor . . . . Mr. Robert W. Smilie

This handbook was originally prepared by the Convair Division of General Dynamics Corporation under contract to NASA and was identified as N68-28783. This book is part of a series of books, commonly know as the General Dynamics Series, that has been the basis of many industrial NDT training programs for over 20 years.

Now, after several decades of widespread use, the entire series has undergone a major revision. The revised material no longer concentrates on applications in the aerospace industry, but instead, covers a wider range of industrial applications and discusses the newest techniques and applications.

Mr. Robert W. Smilie has been the principal author of the revised material in this text. Using his nondestructive testing experiences in several industries, including work at the EPRI NDE Center, he has updated the text to better suit the entry-level technician/engineer.

TABLE OF CONTENTS

Page

PREFACE

Programmed Instruction Handbook - Ultrasonic Testing PI-4, (3 volumes) is one of a series of training handbooks designed for **self-study** applications. The programmed instruction format allows the student to learn the material when a formal classroom setting is not available.

This Programmed Instruction Handbook is also very helpful when used prior to, or in conjunction with, the **Classroom Training Handbook** CT-4, Ultrasonic Testing. The instructor can make assignments in the classroom handbook and, as a supplement, the student can read corresponding information in this self-study handbook to provide a more structured approach for individual learning.

This **Programmed Instruction Handbook** presents essentially the same entry-level material as in the Classroom Training Handbook. However, this **self-study format** provides self-evaluation quiz questions at the end of each chapter and at the end of the book. A score of 80% or better on the Self-Test will indicate the student's understanding of the basic Level I concepts on this subject.

Other **Programmed Instruction Handbooks** in the series include:

PI-1	Introduction to Nondestructive Testing
PI-2	Liquid Penetrant Testing
PI-3	Magnetic Particle Testing
PI-5	Eddy Current Testing
PI-6	Radiographic Testing

CHAPTER 1

ULTRASONIC EQUIPMENT AND TECHNIQUE SELECTION

So far in your study of ultrasonic testing, you have learned the basic principles of ultrasound, its generation, and how it can be used to detect and locate discontinuities in materials of various types and composition. You are also familiar with the equipment and methods of presenting ultrasonic testing results.

Before going into the application of ultrasonics, it would be well to review the techniques covered thus far. You will recall that ultrasonic equipment was placed into two general categories: pulse-echo and through-transmission.

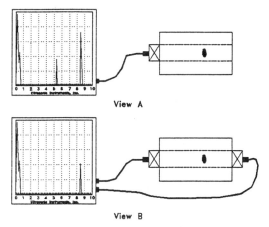

View A

View B

The views above illustrate the two general categories of ultrasonic testing that we have discussed. Which view illustrates the principles of pulse-echo testing?

View A . . . . **Page 1-2**

View B . . . . **Page 1-4**

Right—View A best illustrates the principles of pulse-echo testing.

Now, let's recall what is meant by the term "pulse echo." In pulse-echo testing, we found that pulses of ultrasound are generated by the instrument and introduced into a material, usually by a single transducer. The ultrasound travels through the material and is reflected from the opposite side of the material back to the transducer. The transducer converts the sound vibrations of the reflected pulse to electrical pulses which are typically displayed on a cathode-ray tube (CRT).

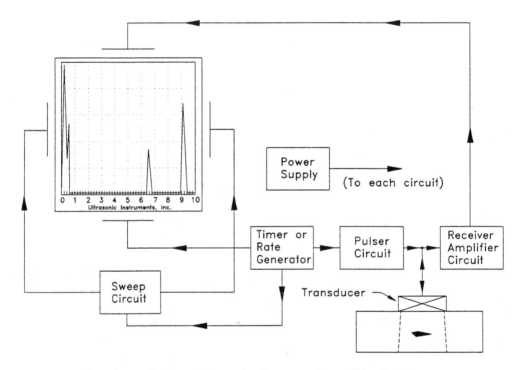

A—scan Pulse Echo Instrument — Block Diagram

Select the statement below which most nearly describes the nature of the ultrasound introduced into the material.

Short pulses of ultrasonic energy .... **Page 1-5**

Continuous ultrasonic energy .... **Page 1-6**

Correct again—the through-transmission system uses separate transducers for transmitting and receiving ultrasonic energy.

You will recall that ultrasonic testing may be further classified as either contact or immersion testing. The decision to use contact testing or immersion testing depends on many factors, all of which you will learn in this Volume. Now let's take a look at contact testing as illustrated below.

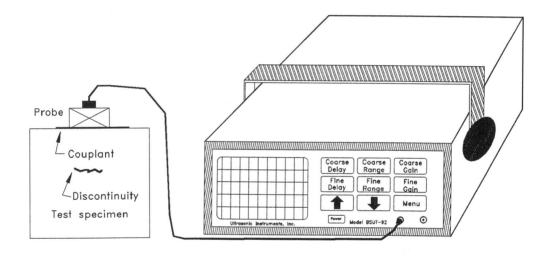

In contact pulse-echo testing, three things are required: (1) a test system, (2) a suitable couplant, and (3) a test specimen. In this case, the transducer is brought into contact with the test specimen, with the couplant between the transducer and the specimen.

Contact testing means that the:

transducer is placed directly in contact with the test
specimen .... **Page 1-8**
transducer is coupled through a thin layer of couplant
to the test specimen .... **Page 1-10**

Your selection of View B as the best illustration of pulse-echo testing is incorrect. View B shows the *through-transmission* system using two transducers; one as a transmitter and one as a receiver. More about through-transmission later.

First, let's take another look at View A.

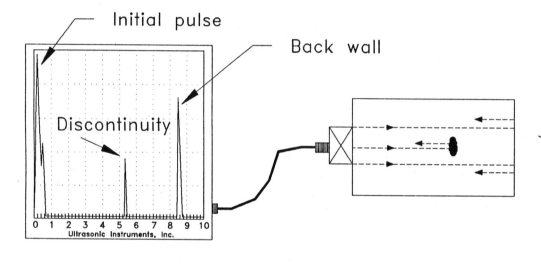

View A

Didn't we learn that the pulse-echo system uses *reflected* energy to determine the presence of discontinuities? Yes. Now, doesn't View A best illustrate this principle? Of course.

Turn back to page 1-2.

Good. You remembered that when using the pulse-echo technique, short pulses of ultrasonic energy are introduced into the test specimen.

The through-transmission system operates on the principle of transmitting ultrasound waves through a test specimen with one transducer and receiving with a second transducer as illustrated.

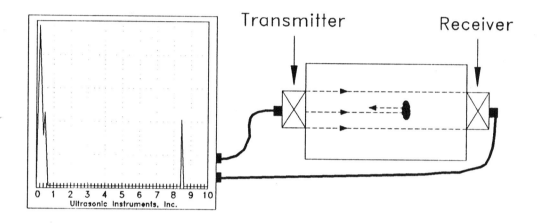

The transmitted sound can be either continuous or pulsed. The presence of a discontinuity is indicated by a reduction in the magnitude of sound energy reaching the receiving transducer.

Through-transmission ultrasonic testing:

Incorrect. Your selection of continuous ultrasonic energy as best describing the nature of the sound introduction into the material by a pulse-echo instrument indicates that you do not understand the meaning of the term "pulse echo."

If the transmitting probe is transmitting, how can it receive? It can't! Therefore, if you are introducing continuous ultrasound into the test specimen, any reflections that exist will not be "heard" by the instrument. This does not imply that through-transmission testing is continuous. In fact, most of it is not.

As the name implies, the "pulse-echo" technique introduces a *short pulse of energy* into the test specimen. The nature of *the indication received* from the test specimen determines if there are any discontinuities present.

Turn back to page 1-5.

Your selection indicates you did not get the point that separate transducers *are used* in through-transmission testing. Well, separate transducers are used, one on one side of the specimen for transmitting sound energy into the specimen and one on the other side of the specimen as a receiver.

Remember, sound reflections are *not* used in through-transmission testing. The presence of a discontinuity is indicated by a reduction in the magnitude of the ultrasound that passes through the specimen.

Turn back to page 1-3.

You think contact testing means placing the transducer in direct contact with the test specimen. You are incorrect.

In Volume I we talked about acoustic impedance and the effect that a large ratio of acoustic impedance has in the transfer of ultrasound energy from one medium to another. If the transducer is placed directly in contact with the test specimen, there is a layer of air between the two surfaces. This air will effectively cause all the sound energy to be reflected back to the transducer since air is such a poor conductor of ultrasound.

Now, if you put a couplant between the two surfaces, a good transfer of sound energy will take place. Remember that a couplant is any substance (such as oil, glycerine, water, etc.) that will fill the space between the transducer and the test specimen and provide a good impedance match between the two.

Turn ahead to page 1-10.

There are many advantages to the immersion technique as compared to contact testing. For the moment though, the important difference to remember is that both the transducer and the test specimen are immersed in the couplant.

Select the best completion for the following statement. In this type of immersion testing, in addition to the liquid in the tank, an oil couplant applied to the face of the transducer:

is not required . . . . **Page 1-11**
is required . . . . **Page 1-13**

Fine. By contact testing we mean the transducer is in contact with the test specimen through a thin layer of couplant.

Now that we have reviewed the basic elements required for contact testing, let's continue by describing immersion testing.

In one type of immersion testing, the test specimen and the transducer are placed in a liquid (usually water) contained in a large tank. The liquid acts as the couplant in the transfer of sound energy from the transducer to the test specimen. The set-up for this type of immersion testing is illustrated below.

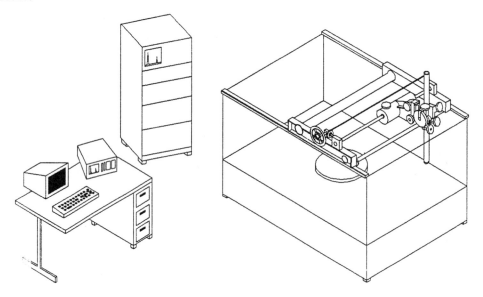

Turn back to page 9.

That's right. An oil couplant is *not* required, since the liquid in the immersion tank acts as the couplant. There are many other significant differences between contact and immersion testing. However, as long as you understand that the primary difference is the couplant, you are ready to proceed to the application of the techniques that have been developed for testing materials of various compositions and shapes.

Ultrasonic testing is particularly adaptable to the determination of the structural integrity of materials. Major applications are in the *detection of discontinuities* in raw stock and finished articles and in *thickness measurements*. The advantages of ultrasonic testing include:

- High sensitivity that permits detection of small defects.
- Great penetrating power that allows examination of a variety of thick materials.
- Accuracy in determination of discontinuity location, position, shape, and size estimation.
- Readily accommodates automated testing.
- Accessibility to only one surface of the test specimen is required (contact pulse-echo testing).
- Portability (contact testing primarily).

From the above listing of the advantages of ultrasonic testing, it is apparent that it has the potential for a variety of applications.

You could say that ultrasonic testing:

**replaces most other nondestructive testing methods . . . Page 1-12
is another nondestructive testing method that may
be selected, depending upon the requirements of the
test to be performed** . . . . **Page 1-14**

Wrong. Even though it is a very versatile method and has capabilities that may not be found in other methods, ultrasonic testing does *not* replace other nondestructive testing methods. Rather it is used in conjunction with other methods to obtain the most knowledge about the specimen under test.

The discussion on the limitations of ultrasonic testing which follows will clear up this point.

Turn ahead to page 1-14.

No—in immersion testing, with the test specimen and transducer both immersed in a tank of liquid, it is not necessary to apply an oil couplant to the face of the transducer. The liquid in the tank provides the necessary coupling between the transducer and test specimen.

The purpose of a couplant is to exclude air from the space between the transducer and the surface of the test specimen and to obtain a better match of acoustic impedance. The liquid in an immersion testing tank performs the function of allowing ultrasound to travel into the test specimen.

Turn back to page 1-11.

Good. You have readily determined that ultrasonic testing is only one of a number of nondestructive testing methods that may be selected. The selection of the test method depends upon the requirements of the test to be performed.

As with all nondestructive testing methods, there are also certain limitations to the use of ultrasonics. Test conditions that may limit the application of ultrasonic techniques are:

● Unfavorable geometry of the test specimen (i.e., size, contour, part complexity, and orientation of defects).
● Undesirable internal structure (i.e., grain size, porosity, inclusion content, or finely-dispersed precipitates).
● Pre-cleaning or post-cleaning of the specimen.

These factors affect the "defect detectability" of the testing technique. "Defect detectability" of the article under test is determined largely by the sensitivity and resolution of the test system used. You will recall that sensitivity is defined as the ability of the test system to detect a small discontinuity at a given distance in a test specimen. And resolution is defined as the ability of the test system to distinguish between indications from discontinuities or reflectors that occur close together.

Given two pulse-echo test systems, system number one is capable of distinguishing between indications from discontinuities that are 1/4 inch (6.3 mm) apart in depth while system number two can only distinguish a difference in indications from discontinuities that are 1/2 inch (12.7 mm) apart in depth. **System number one can be said to have the best:**

sensitivity . . . . **Page 1-16**
resolution . . . . **Page 1-18**

Right—the CRT pattern shown in View A indicates that another method of nondestructive testing should be contemplated as a complement or supplement to ultrasonics. Any discontinuities that might be in the test specimen would not be distinguishable because of the excessive "noise" or "grass" appearing on the screen. High attenuation and rough surface conditions are also factors that can limit the use of an ultrasonic test.

The pulse-echo system is the most widely used in ultrasonic testing. An important advantage of the pulse-echo system is that it does not have the problem of orientation or alignment between separate transducers as does through-transmission testing. One transducer acts as both the transmitter and receiver of the sound energy, and the reflections from discontinuities provide specific information as to discontinuity location, relative size and distance from the examination surface of the test specimen.

The through-transmission system also has certain advantages. Its main advantage is better near surface resolution as a result of using separate transducers for the transmission and reception of sound energy. This advantage allows the detection of discontinuities lying just below the surface of a test specimen that would be difficult to find otherwise. We must remember, though, that dual-element contact probes were designed to provide good near surface resolution in much the same manner.

Turn ahead to page 1-17.

Incorrect. System number one has the best *resolution*. You missed the distinguishing features of the differences in definition of resolution and sensitivity.

Again, sensitivity is the ability of the system to detect the minute amount of sound energy reflected from a small discontinuity in a test specimen at a given distance.

Resolution is the ability of the test system to distinguish between indications from reflectors that are close together in the test specimen.

Turn ahead to page 1-18.

Attenuation is a lesser problem in through-transmission, since the sound energy has to travel in only one direction through the test specimen. This makes it possible for us to test thicker specimens than if we were using pulse-echo.

The principal limitation of through-transmission testing is the requirement that the transmitting and receiving transducers have to be precisely oriented or aligned on the test specimen for proper results. Also, the use of separate transducers doubles the problems of surface alignment, roughness, and couplant.

Which of the following would you select to test a specimen if you needed to know the location, depth and relative size of any discontinuities found?

Through-transmission .... **Page 1-20**
Pulse-echo .... **Page 1-22**

An excellent choice. The resolution of system number one is the better of the two. It can better discern between indications from reflectors that are closely spaced.

Another important factor affecting defect detectability is the signal-to-noise ratio (SNR) of the test system/article combination. SNR is defined as the capability of the test system to discriminate, based on amplitude, between discontinuity signals and undesired signals of either electrical or acoustical nature. These unwanted signals could be the result of unfavorable geometry of the test specimen or its internal structure (i.e., grain size, porosity, and inclusion content). Signals appearing as spurious indications are called "grass" or "noise."

Which of the following CRT patterns indicates a poor SNR and suggests that another method of nondestructive testing be considered?

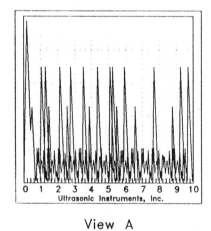

View A   View B

View A . . . . **Page 1-15**
View B . . . . **Page 1-19**

Incorrect—the display in *View A* indicates a poor SNR and suggests another method of nondestructive testing be considered (e.g., radiography, magnetic particle, etc.). View B represents a favorable test system response.

You'll recall that spurious indications and noise were briefly discussed in Volume I where the various displays were presented. We found from these patterns that it was easy to have a discontinuity go undetected because of the many multiple reflections appearing in the display. Spurious indications could also be mistaken for discontinuities. Therefore, in cases where these conditions are present, another method of nondestructive testing should be appraised as a complement or supplement to ultrasonics.

Turn back to page 1-15.

You selected the incorrect answer. Through-transmission will *not* give you the depth of a discontinuity. For this reason, *pulse-echo* would be best.

Turn ahead to page 1-22.

One of the main advantages of contact testing is its flexibility. Instrument portability allows the test equipment to be taken to the material or products to be tested. Other advantages of contact testing include the following.

- A minimum of test instrumentation and accessories is required.
- Its capability for surface wave testing.
- It can be automated.
- Its ability to test large specimens.
- It is relatively inexpensive.

From a review of the advantages of contact testing, it is obvious that this technique, in general, does *not* lend itself to automatic scanning and recording.

True . . . . **Page 1-23**
False . . . . **Page 1-25**

Excellent—you selected the correct answer. Pulse-echo would be the best technique to use if you needed to know the depth of any discontinuities found. You remembered it is impossible to determine a discontinuity's depth when using through-transmission testing.

Let us now take a look at some of the advantages of the contact technique of ultrasonic testing.

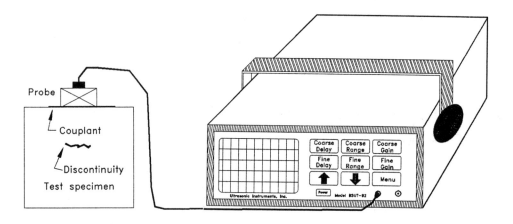

Turn back to page 1-21.

From your selection of a "true" answer, it is apparent that you think contact testing *does not* lend itself to automatic scanning and recording. Sorry, your selection is incorrect.

In this technique, the transducer can be scanned over the test specimen by utilizing automated portable contact scanners. It must be said, however, that in certain high-speed production-line-type applications, contact testing would NOT be the better choice.

Turn ahead to page 1-25.

The principal advantages of immersion testing are:

- The use of higher test frequencies which leads to high scanning speeds and higher sensitivity to small discontinuities.
- The ease at which transducer angulation can be varied.
- Ability to scan irregularly-shaped articles and/or test specimens with rough surfaces.
- Better near surface resolution.

Does immersion testing lend itself to automatic scanning and recording as in a production line process?

Yes . . . . **Page 1-27**
No . . . . **Page 1-29**

Correct. In the contact testing technique, the transducer can be scanned over the specimen and the indications automatically recorded. This instrumentation will be discussed later. It must be said, however, that in certain high-speed production-line-type applications, contact testing would NOT be the better choice.

Limitations of Contact Testing

* The difficulty in maintaining uniform acoustical coupling between the test surface and the transducer that contributes to loss of sensitivity in the testing system and nonuniform test results.

* The requirement for reasonably smooth surfaces in order that there be a maximum transfer of ultrasonic energy to the test specimen.

* Post-examination cleaning of couplants from test specimens, if required.

* The presence of the initial pulse in the display when using single-element probes. This limits near surface resolution.

* The lack of ability to readily vary transducer angle as is possible in immersion testing. (In an extremely limited number of cases this is possible through the use of a variable-angle transducer.)

Analysis of the limitations to the contact testing technique indicates the main disadvantage is:

lack of near surface resolution .... **Page 1-26**
difficulty in maintaining uniform acoustical coupling .... **Page 1-28**

One of the disadvantages of contact testing is the lack of near surface resolution, which means that discontinuities on the examination surface or just beneath the examination surface cannot be detected. This area of the test specimen is often obscured by the initial pulse of the test system when using single-element probes.

However, the *main disadvantage* is the difficulty in maintaining uniform acoustical coupling between the face of the transducer and the surface of the test specimen. The sensitivity of the testing system and the test results will vary if the operator does not maintain uniform pressure on the transducer while it is in contact with the test specimen. This also affects the thickness of the couplant layer.

Turn ahead to page 1-28.

Correct. Immersion testing *does* lend itself to automated scanning and recording such as a production line process. Automated scanning and recording simply requires the addition of a motor-driven carriage with an automated indexing mechanism for scanning the specimen and a printer or other output device.

We also find that immersion testing has certain limitations. These limitations are:

- A large number of accessories are required.
- The size of some specimens will not permit immersion in a tank.
- It is relatively expensive.
- It is often highly specialized.

Suppose we had a small specimen at some field location that we wanted to test ultrasonically. Which technique would you most likely select?

Contact technique . . . . **Page 1-30**
Immersion technique . . . . **Page 1-32**

Excellent. You have correctly selected the difficulty encountered in maintaining uniform acoustical coupling between the surface of the test specimen and transducer as a main disadvantage of contact testing. The lack of uniform acoustical coupling is caused primarily by the operator not being able to maintain a constant pressure on the transducer which also affects the couplant layer thickness. These combined problems, along with excess surface roughness, reduce the sensitivity of the testing system and will cause nonuniform test results.

Now let's take a look at the advantages and limitations of immersion testing.

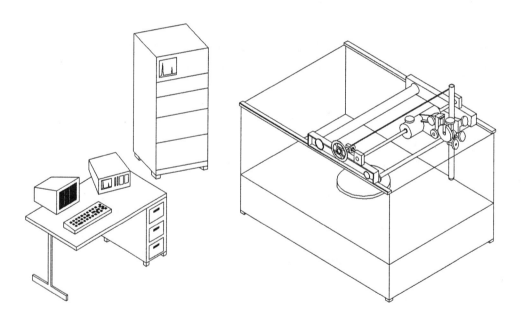

Turn back to page 1-24.

You are incorrect when you say that immersion testing does not lend itself to automatic scanning and recording. It *does*. In fact, many automated ultrasonic systems use the immersion technique or a variation thereof.

Let's recall the typical test setup used in immersion testing. It includes the test instrument, an immersion tank, and a manipulator supported by the carriage. The transducer is mounted in the lower end of a scanner tube in the manipulator.

Now, by using a motor-driven carriage with an automatic indexing mechanism in place of a manually-operated unit, can a transducer be set up to automatically scan a test specimen? Sure it can. In addition, a recording can be made of the scanning operation using a printer or other output device.

Turn back to page 1-27.

Very good. Due to its portability, contact testing would most likely be the best technique to use when testing in the field. The immersion technique would be better in the laboratory or on a production line, depending on the test requirements.

As you can see from the preceding discussions, there are many variables to be considered in ultrasonic testing, some of which are controlled by the operator and some by the inspection problem itself.

In the selection of equipment, the operator determines the type of instrument to be used and the type and size of transducer to be employed. Once the equipment has been selected, the operator controls all the variables of equipment operation. Furthermore, the equipment operation variables can be classed as those relating to *technique* or *control settings*.

Variables in "technique" are those selections which are possible relative to the coupling method, the sequence of scanning the test specimen, and the procedures and acceptance criteria used.

Variables in "control settings" are relative to the test instrument and include the selection of operating frequency, pulse length, and sensitivity. Improper selection of any of the operator-controlled variables can affect the results obtained from the test.

Among the variables controlled by the ultrasonic operator are:

Incorrect. A test specimen may be of an infinite number of shapes and sizes. If you were the ultrasonic test operator and you modified the shape of the specimen before making a test, you would be approaching the field of destructive testing rather than nondestructive testing.

The operator cannot modify the shape of a specimen; however, the operator can adjust the test instrument controls to reduce undesirable effects. In Volume II you learned that most ultrasonic instruments are provided with internal electronic control circuits that enable the operator to vary the CRT presentation or instrument indication to obtain a desired response.

Turn ahead to page 1-36.

Incorrect. The immersion technique does *not* lend itself very well to field testing. This is due largely to the number of accessories and bulky equipment required—it is not very portable.

On the other hand, we find the contact technique well suited for field testing. We do not have to contend with the immersion tank, carriage, manipulator, etc. Remember, portability is one of the main advantages of contact testing.

Turn back to page 1-30.

Your analysis was faulty this time. The acceptance criteria to be used *is not* determined by operator judgment.

Reference blocks are used to establish discontinuity size. We will find that the type of test block, material, etc., is prescribed in the test procedure. It is the responsibility of the operator to evaluate indications from the test specimen with reference to the artificial discontinuity indications provided by the standard reference blocks or reference specimens prescribed.

Turn ahead to page 1-38.

You are correct. The operator controls the selection of the transducer, equipment and operation of the equipment. A lot of responsibility for success or failure of the tests still depends on the operator.

The second set of variables in any ultrasonic testing situation are those controlled by the inspection problem. These variables are the properties of the test specimen and discontinuity conditions that may exist.

Properties of a test specimen that will affect a particular ultrasonic test are:

- The sound velocity within the specimen.
- The acoustic impedance of the material.
- The shape and surface condition of the specimen.
- The sound attenuation and "noise" level within the specimen.

Discontinuity conditions that may exist in a test specimen vary over a wide range. Their effect on a test situation depends on:

- The sound-path distance to the discontinuity.
- The size and shape of the discontinuity.
- The acoustic impedance of the discontinuity relative to that of the test specimen.
- The orientation of the discontinuity with respect to the specimen's examination surface.

Given a particular test specimen, which of the following may be modified by the operator?

Shape of the specimen .... **Page 1-31**
Adjustment of the test instrument .... **Page 1-36**

By turning to this page you indicate that you think good test documentation will serve as a crutch and reduce the need for training of operators of ultrasonic equipment. Look at the requirements again - it merely serves as a starting point, sets up the general requirements for the test, and provides a reference point for evaluating discontinuity indications from the test specimen.

One of the most important requirements of an operator of ultrasonic equipment is the ability to evaluate the indications received from a discontinuity. This ability can only come from training and experience.

Turn ahead to page 1-40.

Excellent. An ultrasonic test operator can adjust only the test instrument controls to obtain a better response or presentation. About the only modification an operator can make to a test specimen is to modify its surface condition. With proper authorization, you may sometimes smooth the specimen surface if it is so rough that ultrasonic testing is impractical.

Now that you understand that there are many variables that must be considered in performing ultrasonic testing successfully, let's take a look at some of the general requirements for successful testing. These are:

- A clear definition of the test to be performed.
- The presence of well-trained properly-supervised operators. Operators must also possess a basic understanding of materials and their processing.
- An adequate supply of standard reference blocks or reference specimens to be used for comparison to test specimens.
- A good test procedure.
- Realistic acceptance standards.

Key factors for successful ultrasonic testing is to have well-trained operators and to provide these operators with a test procedure and acceptance standards that clearly define the extent of discontinuities that may be tolerated in a test specimen.

From an analysis of the above general requirements, what would you say determines the type of acceptance criteria to be used in evaluating discontinuity indications?

The standards are determined by operator judgment ... Page 1-33
The standards are stated in the test procedure .... Page 1-38

You are partially correct. The operator *does not* have any control over the test specimen. The operator's assignment to perform an ultrasonic test on a particular specimen or group of specimens is a fixed quantity and cannot be controlled by the operator. The operator does have control over the transducer selected. Re-read page 1-30 then turn to page 1-34.

Excellent. You haven't been told anything about acceptance standards yet, but you have correctly determined that the type of standard reference block or reference specimen to be used will be prescribed in the test procedure.

General requirements for test procedures are:

- Operator qualifications.
- Instrumentation, equipment, and system details.
- Testing technique.
- Scanning technique.
- Reference standards - a requirement that discontinuities be compared to reflections returned from equipment calibrated previously with ultrasonic reference blocks.
- Acceptance criteria - ultrasonic quality levels are provided by acceptance standards or codes.

It appears that a good test procedure and its governing code provides a lot of detail about an ultrasonic test to be performed.

Would you say that this test documentation reduces the need for operator training or that it has no effect on the need for training?

Reduces need for operator training . . . . **Page 1-35**
Has no effect on operator training requirement . . . . **Page 1-40**

Your selection is not correct. We cannot base all our calibrations on a 3/64-inch (1.2 mm) FBH in a steel reference block. What if we are examining a weld in an aluminum pipe or a composite aircraft wing?

What is really desired during calibration is to determine the magnitude of the reflection obtained from a simulated discontinuity in the appropriate test or reference block.

Turn ahead to page 1-42.

That is right. Regardless of how good the test documentation is, we still have a need for thorough operator training. No written material will substitute for the judgment required in evaluating the discontinuity indications that may be expected when submitting test specimens to ultrasonic testing.

Once a determination has been made of the correct technique of conducting the test (contact or immersion), and the equipment selected (pulse-echo or through-transmission), it is necessary to assure that the test instrument is calibrated against ultrasonic test blocks *before* proceeding with the test.

When acceptance of material is based on rigid ultrasonic test standards, very close attention must be paid to the calibration of test instruments to assure that accurate test results will be obtained.

Calibration of ultrasonic systems is based on reflections from:

a 3/64-inch (1.2 mm) FBH in a steel reference block . . . . **Page 1-39**
reflectors as specified in the test procedure . . . . **Page 1-42**

At times it may be necessary to fabricate test blocks when standard reference test blocks are not available in the same material as that of the test specimen. In some cases, a portion of the test specimen is removed and artificial discontinuities are introduced. This can be by drilling carefully-machined flat-bottomed holes at certain depths, or by fabricating notches or inducing cracks which will produce artificial discontinuity indications. Calibration blocks may also contain laminations, side-drilled holes or any combination of these reflectors depending on the intended application.

Is the following statement true or false? Test blocks made from carbon steel bar stock would be suitable for calibrating the test instrument prior to performing tests on a carbon steel casting.

True . . . . **Page 1-43**
False . . . . **Page 1-45**

Excellent. The principal method for calibration of test systems is based on reflectors, natural or artificial, as specified in the test procedure.

In Volume II you learned that standard reference blocks are provided with precisely-machined holes of varying dimensions and depths. You also learned that artificial discontinuities are often fabricated for the purpose of providing simulated discontinuities for calibration. In this Volume you have learned that test blocks are prescribed as standards against which to compare discontinuities in test specimens.

Ultrasonic test procedures for the various tests will prescribe the test block and discontinuity type and size that is to be used as a reference. Since these test blocks often have ideal geometry and surface conditions, most discontinuities in the test specimen whose reflection amplitude is equal to the reflection from the test hole will tend to be *larger* than the dimensions of the calibration reference. Recall that the test article itself may cause variations in the amplitude of the CRT indications due to factors such as grain structure and attenuation.

Test blocks used for calibration should be similar to the test specimen in the following respects:

- Alloy content (or material specification).
- Heat treatment.
- Degree of hot or cold working due to forging, rolling, or extruding.
- Temperature.
- Surface condition.

Turn back to page 1-41.

By selecting a "true" answer you are indicating that you think discontinuity indications from a carbon steel bar stock and a carbon steel casting would be very nearly the same. If the equipment is calibrated using test blocks of carbon steel bar stock, discontinuity indications from the casting *could* be correctly interpreted.

This answer *could* be considered correct under certain conditions, but usually there will be large errors in evaluating discontinuity indications from the casting. The material specifications, and most likely the ultrasonic characteristics, are *not* similar. Therefore, your "True" selection must be considered wrong because, under practical test conditions, you could not be sure that the comparison between the bar stock and the casting would reveal equal discontinuity indications.

Turn ahead to page 1-45.

Next, the test specimen discontinuity is rechecked and its amplitude compared with the amplitude of the reflection from the test block. It is found to have a response of 66% FSH at a sound path of approximately 2 inches (50.8 mm).

The discontinuity detected and sized in this test article is:

unacceptable . . . . **Page 1-46**
acceptable . . . . **Page 1-47**

Right. If test blocks of carbon steel bar stock are used for calibrating the test system and tests are performed on carbon steel castings, the indications from discontinuities in the test specimen may have no relationship in size to the indications received from simulated discontinuities in the test blocks. This is because of variations in the internal structure of the two materials and therefore acoustical properties.

Consider now a practical example of the use of calibration blocks. Suppose the ultrasonic procedure requires that discontinuity indications in excess of the response from a 3/64-inch (1.2 mm) flat-bottomed hole at the sound path of the discontinuity be cause for rejection of the specimen.

Assume that, while testing a specimen with a contact pulse-echo system, we obtained an indication which revealed a discontinuity at a sound-path distance of 2 inches (50.8 mm) into the test specimen.

We would then select a test block of a material similar to the test specimen with a 3/64-inch (1.2 mm) flat-bottomed hole drilled to a depth such that the flat bottom of the hole is approximately 2 inches (50.8 mm) from the examination surface of the block.

Using the instrument sensitivity (gain) control, we would then adjust the response from the test block to display the flat-bottomed hole indication to 60% FSH on the CRT.

Turn to the previous page.

Excellent. The discontinuity indication is greater in amplitude and therefore greater in relative size to the maximum acceptable indication. In accordance with the test procedure, this discontinuity now becomes a defect or flaw and should be recorded as such on the examination report.

In summation, you have learned in this chapter that in the selection of an ultrasonic test system and technique:

● Ultrasonic testing has its advantages and limitations with respect to other methods of nondestructive testing.
● System and technique selection depend largely on the test environment and the test results required.
● Many variables must be considered, some of which are operator controlled and some controlled by the inspection problem itself.
● The particular requirements of a test are set forth in the test procedure.
● Reference (calibration) blocks are used to evaluate discontinuities.
● Calibration is a must in evaluating discontinuity indications.

Also of great importance is the calibration and alignment of the circuits within an ultrasonic test instrument. Normally an instrument must bear a current and valid periodic calibration sticker before it can be considered acceptable for performance of a test. However, the details of this calibration are beyond the scope of this handbook.

Turn ahead to page 1-48 for a review of what you have learned in this chapter.

Your "acceptable" selection is not correct. The test procedure required the rejection of any discontinuity that produced a response in excess of 60% FSH at approximately the same sound path distance. Our calibration 3/64-inch (1.2 mm) FBH reflector produced a 60% FSH response at a sound path of 2 inches (50.8 mm). The detected discontinuity produced a 66% FSH response at the same sound-path distance. It is therefore unacceptable for continued service.

Turn back to page 1-46.

CHAPTER REVIEW

_____ 1. In pulse-echo ultrasonic testing, _____ pulses of sound energy are transmitted into a test specimen.

    A.   short
    B.   long
    C.   continuous
    D.   leading

_____ 2. The pulse-echo system provides specific information as to a discontinuity's _____ and its _____ from the test specimen's examination surface.

    A.   color, location
    B.   style, depth
    C.   color, location
    D.   size, sound-path distance

_____ 3. Through-transmission testing uses _____ transducers.

    A.   three
    B.   two
    C.   one
    D.   seven

_____ 4. The technique of ultrasonic testing where the transducer is placed on the test specimen with a thin couplant separating them is called:

    A. contact testing.
    B. immersion testing.
    C. through-pulsation testing.
    D. pulsed testing.

_____ 5. The technique of ultrasonic testing where the test specimen and transducer are placed in treated water is called _____ testing.

    A. pulsed
    B. pulse-echo
    C. immersion
    D. through-echo

_____ 6. The most widely used applications of the ultrasonic techniques are in _____ measurement and _____ detection.

    A. lamination, burst
    B. burst, thickness
    C. discontinuity, lamination
    D. thickness, discontinuity

_____   7.   Defect detectability is largely dependent on the _____ and _____ of the test system in use.

A.   height, weight
B.   size, type
C.   sensitivity, resolution
D.   probe, computer compatibility

_____   8.   The best near surface resolution can be obtained using the _____ system.

A.   pulse-echo
B.   through-transmission
C.   through-pulsation
D.   Ultrasonics Incorporated

_____   9.   To determine the depth and specific size of a discontinuity, we would use the _____ system.

A.   X-ray
B.   penetrant
C.   through-transmission
D.   pulse-echo

_____   10.   The problem of transducer alignment is a principal disadvantage of _____ testing.

A.   through-transmission
B.   pulse-echo
C.   high-speed
D.   thickness

11. Attenuation is a _____ problem in through-transmission testing than in pulse-echo testing.

A. lesser
B. greater

12. Compared to the contact technique, the immersion technique has a _____ sensitivity to small discontinuities.

A. lower
B. constant
C. higher

13. Transducer angulation is easier using the _____ technique.

A. contact
B. through-pulsation
C. immersion
D. through-transmission

14. Test specimen size is a limiting factor in _____ testing.

A. contact-immersion
B. contact
C. through-transmission
D. immersion

15. Variables in an ultrasonic testing system that are controlled by the operator are equipment:

A.   selection and operation.
B.   coupling and scanning sequence.
C.   test procedures and scanning sequence.
D.   acceptance criteria and test procedures.

16. Given a test specimen of a certain size, shape, acoustic impedance, surface condition, and discontinuity properties, only the _____ (with proper authorization) can be modified by the ultrasonic operator.

A.   material specification
B.   surface condition
C.   discontinuity properties
D.   shape

17. Assume you are performing an ultrasonic test. The _____ prescribes the type of reference block or reference specimen that will be used to compare with discontinuity indications in the test article.

A.   scanning sequence
B.   surface condition
C.   test procedure
D.   instrument manufacturer

_____ 18. Calibration of ultrasonic instruments can be based on reflections from flat-bottomed _____ in standard reference (test) blocks.

    A. discontinuities
    B. cracks
    C. laminations
    D. holes

_____ 19. If a wrought steel plate is being tested by ultrasonics, the reference blocks used for calibrating the test instrument should be made of:

    A. wrought steel.
    B. aluminum.
    C. cast steel.
    D. any wrought metal.

_____ 20. Assume that a discontinuity indication is 80% FSH from a test specimen. The magnitude of the indication from a 5/64-inch (2.0 mm) flat-bottomed hole at the same approximate sound-path distance is also 80% FSH. It can be assumed that the size of the actual discontinuity is _____ the flat-bottomed hole.

    A. smaller than
    B. the same size as
    C. larger than
    D. not comparable to

21. The ultrasonic testing category in which discontinuities are indicated by a reduction or loss of transmitted energy in the test specimen is called:

A.   pulse-echo.
B.   through-pulsation.
C.   through-transmission.
D.   immersion echo.

22. Difficulty in maintaining uniform acoustical coupling between the test specimen and the transducer is a disadvantage of _____ testing.

A.   through-pulsation
B.   contact
C.   through-transmission
D.   digital thickness gauge

23. The most widely used ultrasonic test category is:

A.   through-pulsation.
B.   pulse-echo.
C.   pulse-through.
D.   immersion.

24. Cracks and notches can be used for calibration, should the test procedure (and application) allow it.

A.   True
B.   False

Turn to the next page for answers to these review questions.

ANSWERS TO REVIEW QUESTIONS
FOR CHAPTER 1

Question & Answer		Reference Page(s)
1.	A	1-5
2.	D	1-15
3.	B	1-5
4.	A	1-3
5.	C	1-10
6.	D	1-11
7.	C	1-14
8.	B	1-15
9.	D	1-17, 1-22
10.	A	1-17
11.	A	1-17
12.	C	1-24
13.	C	1-24
14.	D	1-27
15.	A	1-34
16.	B	1-36
17.	C	1-38
18.	D	1-42
19.	A	1-45
20.	C	1-42

Turn to the next page.

Question & Answer		Reference Page(s)
21.	C	1-5
22.	B	1-25
23.	B	1-15
24.	A	1-41

Turn to the next page and begin Chapter 2.

CHAPTER 2

PULSE-ECHO/THROUGH-TRANSMISSION TESTING USING THE CONTACT TECHNIQUE

In Chapter 1 we reviewed the basic system and techniques used in ultrasonic testing. You learned that each has its advantages and limitations depending on the existing test conditions. You learned of many variables that must be considered and the importance and use of test documentation. At this point in your study of ultrasonic testing you should have a "feel" for selecting the most logical test technique and system required to perform a particular test you have at hand.

Let's take a look now at some of the considerations pertinent to the selection of test equipment for contact testing. We'll assume that you have available to you a wide variety of instruments having a variety of characteristics, and that you have many possibilities in the selection of transducers and display devices. In actual practice this ideal condition in which a wide selection of equipment is available will not often be realized. But to obtain the best test results, it is necessary to consider the capabilities of all the equipment that may be available.

Turn to the next page.

This chapter covers the application of two basic categories used in contact ultrasonic testing. These are:

- Pulse-echo using one transducer as both a transmitter and receiver of sound energy, or separate transducers for each function.
- Through-transmission using separate transducers for transmitting and receiving the sound beam.

From the discussions in Chapter 1 on the advantages and limitations of pulse-echo and through-transmission testing, you learned that the pulse echo system is the most widely used. This is true for two reasons. First, there is no problem of positioning the separate transducers for transmission and reception since these two functions are most often combined into one transducer. Second, reflections from discontinuities provide specific information as to the relative size of a discontinuity and its distance from the examination surface of the test specimen.

Shown below is an illustration of through-transmission testing.

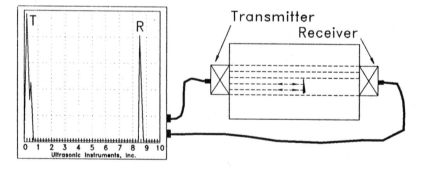

When using through-transmission, are discontinuity indications directly proportional to the amount of sound energy *reflected* by the discontinuity?

Yes .... **Page 2-4**
No .... **Page 2-6**

Very good. When the through-transmission system is used, there is no longer any problem of near surface resolution. Discontinuities just below the surface of the test specimen can be detected. However, due to the limitations previously discussed, through-transmission is not widely used for detection of discontinuities except in special applications.

In contact testing, determination of the proper equipment to be used depends on the following factors:

- Nature, size, orientation, distribution, and number of discontinuities that may be expected in the test specimen.
- Shape, dimensions, and critical areas of the test specimen will determine type of transducer to be used.
- Surface condition, such as smooth or rough, flat or wavy, forged, cast, or rough machined, will determine selection of couplant and test frequency.
- Specimen internal structure may be fine or coarse grained. This will affect attenuation and scattering of the sound beam and will assist in determining the test frequency to be selected.

Turn ahead to page 2-5.

Slow down a bit. You probably didn't read the question carefully enough. We are talking about *through-transmission*.

In through-transmission testing, the pulse at the receiving transducer is NOT directly proportional to the size of the discontinuity. The highest pulse (indication) will be received when there is no discontinuity in the test article. The lowest pulse will be received when the discontinuity is largest.

In fact, then, the receiver indication is *inversely proportional* to the size of the discontinuity.

Turn ahead to page 2-6.

Consideration also should be given to the following performance requirements of an ultrasonic test instrument when making a selection for a particular contact test situation.

- The frequency range capability of the instrument.
- Instrument resolution.
- Linearity of the instrument (the capability of an instrument to display signal amplitude in proportion to amount of reflection from a discontinuity).
- Instrument penetration power (Is sufficient power available to penetrate the test specimen?).
- Instrument sensitivity to give the required indication amplitude.
- Capability for both single- and dual-transducer applications as required.

Select the best completion for the following statement.

Ultrasonic equipment selection is dependent on:

test specimen characteristics only .... **Page 2-7**

the test situation .... **Page 2-9**

That is right.   When using through-transmission the CRT indication is *inversely proportional* to the amount of sound energy reflected by a discontinuity. Total reflection of the sound energy will result in no energy being received by the receiving transducer. If there are no discontinuities in the test specimen, the amplitude of the sound energy received by the receiving transducer will be maximum.

We have also learned that through-transmission testing has certain advantages over pulse-echo testing, such as better near surface resolution and the capability of testing thicker test specimens. We also mentioned another option for improving near surface resolution with contact testing. More on that later.

In through-transmission testing, the receiving transducer does not "see" the reflection from the front surface of the test specimen.

At what minimum sound-path distance in the test specimen do you think the presence of discontinuities can be detected?

A few thousandths of an inch (0.05 mm) . . . . **Page 2-3**
About 1/4 inch (6.3 mm) . . . . **Page 2-8**

You did not select the best answer. It is true that the test specimen plays an important part in the selection of ultrasonic test equipment; however, are not the test results we wish to obtain also an important consideration? Of course. We should know the test requirements as well as the characteristics of the test specimen (i.e., shape, size, surface condition, and internal structure) when selecting ultrasonic equipment.

Turn ahead to page 2-9.

Through-transmission testing can do better than 1/4 inch (6.3 mm). Since in through-transmission testing the part of the specimen immediately below the surface is not obscured by the initial pulse, it is possible to detect the presence of discontinuities that lie *a few thousandths of an inch (0.05 mm)* below the surface when using separate transmitting and receiving transducers.

Turn back to page 2-3.

Excellent. You correctly determined that the selection of ultrasonic test equipment is largely dependent on the *test situation* and not on just the test specimen alone.

Once the test situation is established and the basic test instrument selected, it is important to select the proper frequency to test the material in the test specimen to meet the requirements of the test. It is usually desirable to test at the lowest frequency that will locate specified minimum sizes and types of discontinuities consistently. Because of variations in the structure of materials, it is not possible to specify herein a frequency for all ultrasonic tests of a given material type.

Turn to the next page.

Listed below are the frequency ranges and test applications generally used.

FREQUENCY RANGE	TEST APPLICATION
200 kHz - 1 MHz	CASTINGS: GRAY IRON, NODULAR IRON, AND RELATIVELY COARSE-GRAINED MATERIALS, SUCH AS COPPER AND STAINLESS STEELS.
400 kHz - 5 MHz	CASTINGS: STEEL, ALUMINUM, BRASS, AND OTHER MATERIALS WITH REFINED GRAIN SIZE.
200 kHz - 2.25 MHz	PLASTICS AND PLASTIC-LIKE MATERIALS, SUCH AS SOLID ROCKET PROPELLANTS AND POWDER GRAINS.
1 - 5 MHz	ROLLED PRODUCTS: METALLIC SHEET, PLATE, BARS, AND BILLETS.
2.25 - 10 MHz	DRAWN AND EXTRUDED PRODUCTS: BARS, TUBES, AND SHAPES.
1 - 10 MHz	FORGINGS.
2.25 - 10 MHz	GLASS AND CERAMICS.
1 - 5 MHz	WELDS.
1 - 10 MHz	MAINTENANCE INSPECTION, ESPECIALLY FATIGUE CRACKS.

It should be noted that the term hertz (Hz) is now the universally accepted designation for the measure of frequency instead of cycles per second (cps).

A coarse-grained internal structure in a test specimen will require the selection of a:

high test frequency .... **Page 2-12**
low test frequency .... **Page 2-14**

Your selection of a casting is not correct. A casting will usually have a coarser grain structure than a plate which has been rolled and formed. Grain structure of materials becomes more refined as they go through additional forming processes.

Turn ahead to page 2-13.

Your selection is not correct. A sonic beam of high frequency will be scattered by the coarse grain structure of the test specimen. If the frequency is high enough, the reflections from the scattered beams will probably be such that it will appear that the specimen is defective, while a lower frequency applied to the same specimen will not indicate a rejectable discontinuity. When in doubt about the internal structure of a specimen, the operator should experiment to determine the best frequency to be used for the test.

Turn ahead to page 2-14.

Correct. An aluminum plate will have a finer grain structure than an aluminum casting. Therefore, you would select a lower frequency for testing an aluminum casting.

Before proceeding to the factors that should be considered in the selection of the proper transducer to do the job, let us briefly review the principles that must be considered in selecting the test frequency. These are:

- The highest test frequency will provide the greatest sensitivity for detection of small defects.
- The lowest test frequency will give the power that is necessary to penetrate more deeply into the specimen being tested.

Frequency is one of the factors that determines the ability of a testing system to detect discontinuities close to the surface.

Which of the following will afford the better discontinuity detection based on frequency?

Low test frequencies . . . . **Page 2-15**
High test frequencies . . . . **Page 2-17**

That is correct. A *low* test frequency is required to test a specimen that has a coarse-grained internal structure. A sonic beam of high frequency will be scattered by the grain. Scattering can lead to an interpretation that the specimen is bad. A lower frequency sonic beam may indicate that the specimen is sound.

Not all pieces of steel are the same internally. Forgings, castings, extrusions, and plate all have their own peculiarities of internal grain structure. Some are coarse; others are fine. The characteristics of the internal grain structure are significant when selecting the proper test frequency. For fine-grained materials, a high frequency should be used since a low frequency beam will not "see" the smaller discontinuities. Just the reverse is true for coarse-grained specimens—a lower frequency must be used since a high frequency will cause reflections from the coarse grains. These reflections appear as discontinuity indications in the display.

You will recall that when ultrasound passes through a material, it does so by successive particle displacements. The amount of particle displacement is determined, to a certain extent, by the wavelength of the sound energy. At high frequencies the wavelength is short in relation to the size of the grain in the material and a large amount of the energy is expended as heat since the energy in the wave is insufficient to move the mass of the grains. Thus the sound is prevented from traveling through the specimen. Also, some of the sound energy is reflected back to the transducer, giving false indications of discontinuities.

Which material has the finer grain structure, an aluminum casting or aluminum plate?

Aluminum casting .... **Page 2-11**
Aluminum plate .... **Page 2-13**

Your selection would not give the best resolution in the detection of discontinuities. A *higher* frequency is needed for the best system sensitivity and resolution to detect discontinuities that lie close to the surface.

Lower test frequencies are best where increased power is required to penetrate thick test specimens, and are used when the increased penetration is of more benefit than the location of small discontinuities or the location of discontinuities that lie close to the surface.

Turn ahead to page 2-17.

Suppose now that the material to be tested is large and flat. To test such a specimen you would choose a transducer that covers a large area, either a large, single transducer, or a mosaic of smaller crystals such as could be found in a paintbrush transducer.

If the test is to be made through ridges, shoulders, or other areas restricted in size, you would select a small-diameter transducer.

For a curved surface, a transducer with a contoured wedge would provide maximum contact surface between the transducer and the test specimen.

At a given ultrasonic test frequency, which will give the *largest* beam spread?

A large transducer . . . . **Page 2-18**
A small transducer . . . . **Page 2-20**

Excellent. When you have a choice of low and high test frequencies and want to improve the test system's ability to detect discontinuities, the higher test frequency is the better selection. Combine this benefit with a short pulse length and you will have a combination of factors that will give you the best near surface detection of discontinuities, all other factors held constant.

Now that the problems to be faced in selection of a test frequency are understood, let's proceed to a discussion of the factors to be considered in the selection of transducers. The following factors must be taken into consideration:

- A larger-diameter transducer is required when testing through greater thicknesses.
- Available contact surface area can limit the size of the transducer.
- More beam spread may be desired to detect randomly-oriented discontinuities. Other applications require the narrowest (and straightest) beam possible to minimize reflections from adjacent surfaces of the test specimen.
- A narrower beam is useful for establishing the extremities of large discontinuities which are larger than the total beam spread.
- At any frequency, the larger the crystal, the less the beam spread; the smaller the crystal, the greater the beam spread.
- For a transducer of a given diameter, there is less beam spread at higher frequencies than at lower frequencies.
- Increases in frequency result in increased near zone length.
- The near zone increases substantially (as a squared function) as the probe diameter increases.
- The orientation of the sound beam within the test article (i.e. straight beam versus angle beam).

Turn back to the previous page.

The spread of the beam coming from an ultrasonic transducer is *not* to be considered as proportional to the size of the transducer. Quite the contrary; the *larger* the transducer the *smaller* the beam spread. Just keep in mind that the relationship of beam spread to transducer size is an inverse proportion.

You should have selected "small transducer" as the answer to the question since a small transducer at a given frequency will give the largest beam spread.

Turn ahead to page 2-20.

Excellent. Congratulations on correctly deducing that the refraction angle of the ultrasonic wave in aluminum will be *less* than the refraction angle in steel. You seem to understand the application of Snell's Law.

Now for a review of the considerations in the selection of a transducer for making a test. These are:

- Larger crystals should be used for general testing and whenever the least beam spread and maximum power is required.
- Smaller crystals should be used on uneven surfaces, or when the test surface is too small to permit use of large transducers.
- Selection of an angle beam or straight beam transducer should conform to the testing technique and test article geometry.
- Special contoured wedges should be used when testing curved surfaces.
- For best scanning efficiency in testing large, flat specimens, a paintbrush transducer should be selected, if available.

Turn ahead to page 2-23.

Good. Your answer that a small transducer has a larger beam spread at a given ultrasonic frequency is correct.

Now, let's concern ourselves with the type of discontinuity that the test is expected to detect. The size of the expected discontinuity, its orientation to the examination surface, its distribution in the test specimen, and its distance from the examination surface are important considerations in planning the test.

You will recall that high frequencies are required to locate the smaller discontinuities and to locate discontinuities lying near the examination surface of the specimen. Testing for discontinuities that are at a great distance from the examination surface will require larger transducers than those used for testing for discontinuities closer to the surface.

Suppose you are testing a specimen that is over 10 feet (3 meters) in length. A discontinuity is suspected to lie 10 feet (3 meters) from the examination surface. You have selected 2.25 MHz as the frequency most likely to give the best test results.

With a choice of a 1/2-inch (12.7 mm) or a 1-inch-diameter (25.4 mm) transducer, which should be selected to penetrate to and beyond the suspected discontinuity?

1/2-inch (12.7 mm) transducer . . . . **Page 2-22**
1-inch (25.4 mm) transducer . . . . **Page 2-24**

It appears as though you guessed wrong on this one. Actually, assuming that the angle of incidence remains the same, the angle of refraction in aluminum will be slightly less than the angle of refraction in steel.

When ultrasonic beams are introduced into two different materials using the same angle beam transducer, the angle of refraction in each material is dependent on the velocity of sound in that material. Since the velocity of sound in aluminum is less than the velocity of sound in steel, the angle of refraction in the aluminum will be smaller than the angle of refraction in steel.

The angle beam transducer we are using develops a beam that is angled at 45° to the vertical when the transducer is applied to steel. Since the velocity of sound in aluminum is less than the velocity of sound in steel, the application of the 45° transducer to the aluminum will result in a beam that is angled something *less* than 45° to the vertical.

Turn back to page 2-19.

Did you guess at this one? If so, you guessed wrong. The *1-inch (25.4 mm) transducer* should have been selected. It will produce a higher intensity beam that would be more capable of penetrating the 10-foot (3 meter) distance required for detecting a discontinuity in the suspected area. The 1/2-inch (12.7 mm) transducer would produce a lower intensity beam that most likely would not have sufficient power after traveling the 10 feet (3 meters) to return a measurable reflection.

Turn ahead to page 2-24.

A satisfactory contact test cannot be conducted without use of a suitable couplant between the transducer and the test surface. A couplant, you will remember, is a substance that "wets" the surface and acts to exclude air between the two surfaces.

You learned that for most contact testing applications a thin film of couplant should be used and the thickness between the two surfaces should be uniform. In some applications, where it is not possible to use a liquid couplant, a thin sheet of rubber or plastic may be used. Examples of couplant that may be used are:

- Light machine oil
- Multi-viscosity engine oil
- Water with a wetting agent (common detergent) and corrosion inhibitor
- Water and glycerine with a wetting agent
- Couplants available from couplant manufacturers for most any application
- Glycerin

Turn ahead to page 2-26.

An excellent choice. The 1-inch (25.4 mm) transducer *is* the best selection for the example given. It would produce a higher beam intensity which would more likely return a reflection from a discontinuity at the 10-foot (3 meter) distance if one existed.

The technique to be used in performing the ultrasonic test also has an effect on the selection of the proper transducer. It may be desired that the ultrasonic beam propagate into the test specimen at an angle. In this case, a transducer with a plastic wedge would be selected. The illustration below shows what happens to the sound beam, due to the law of refraction (Snell's Law), when it enters the test specimen at an angle.

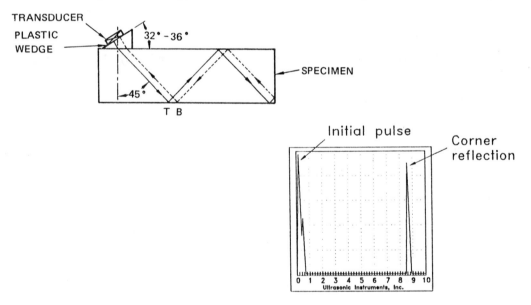

Sound is caused to bounce through the test specimen and reflect back to the transducer along the paths illustrated above.

Turn to the next page.

You will recall that angle beam transducers used for contact testing are available for any desired angle. The common shear wave angles available are for 45°, 60°, and 70° of refraction in steel. Many additional search units are available as catalog items, including longitudinal and bimodal (transmit and receive both shear and longitudinal modes) probes.

If an angle beam transducer will produce a beam angle of 45° in steel and you are to use this transducer for testing aluminum, will the angle of the sound beam in aluminum be greater or less than 45°? Assume that the velocity of sound in aluminum is less than the velocity in steel.

Less than 45° . . . . **Page 2-19**
More than 45° . . . . **Page 2-21**

You learned that a couplant should:

- Be easy to apply
- Not run off the surface too fast
- Be free of bubbles or solid particles
- Be noncorrosive and nontoxic
- Have an acoustic impedance as close as possible to the acoustic impedance of the test specimen (between that of the specimen and transducer)
- Not affect the fabrication operations to follow

Suppose you are conducting a test on a rough vertical surface. Which would be the most suitable couplant?

Engine oil . . . . **Page 2-28**
Water with wetting agent . . . . **Page 2-30**

You sure guessed on this one, didn't you? It doesn't matter how smooth a surface is, a couplant is still required in contact testing.

A thin film of couplant (such as a light oil) will be adequate in the case cited, but a couplant is still needed to exclude air and allow the ultrasonic sound beam to penetrate the test block.

Turn ahead to page 2-31.

A good selection. If testing is to be conducted on a *rough vertical surface* and the selection of couplant to be used is limited to either engine oil or water with a wetting agent, oil is the best couplant to select since it is more viscous and will not run off as quickly.

Once the proper test system has been selected, it will be necessary for the operator to check the horizontal and vertical linearity of the instrument.

These linearities are checked by conducting tests on ultrasonic reference blocks. First, the instrument is connected to the power source, power is turned on, and the equipment is allowed to warm up for the period specified in the manufacturer's instruction book. After warm-up, tests are made on reference blocks of varying thicknesses to determine that adequate artificial discontinuity indications are received from the reflectors and that these indications are, or can be, positioned in the display as instructed in the test procedure.

This procedure is not to be confused with the factory/manufacturer's calibration of the instrument—it merely assures the operator that the instrument is in operating order before proceeding with the test in accordance with the test documentation.

A couplant will NOT be required when making the above checks for instrument linearity since the reference blocks are very precisely machined and the test surface smooth enough that good contact will be made between the transducer and the test surface.

True . . . . **Page 2-27**
False . . . . **Page 2-31**

You selected the wrong answer. Look at the illustration below. You can see what will happen to the sound beam when it strikes the angled rear surface. The beam will reflect at an angle that is equal to the angle of incidence. Since the rear surface is at an angle of 20° to the incident beam, the reflection will be at an angle of 20° and there will be no reflection returning to the transducer for display on the CRT.

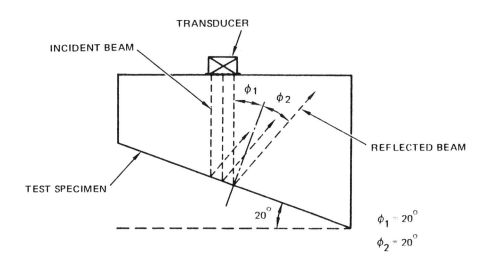

Turn ahead to page 2-32.

Your selection of the couplant is not the best. Water with a wetting agent will provide adequate coupling qualities but will have a tendency to run off the vertical surface too rapidly. Engine oil would be the best of the two couplants in this application. It will provide a film that adheres to the surface long enough for the test to be completed.

Turn back to page 2-28.

"False" is correct. A couplant between a transducer and test surface is required at *all* times, regardless of how smooth the surface is. A very thin layer of couplant will be adequate for the smooth surface involved.

Before conducting a test, you should have a clear idea of the kind and quantity of discontinuities you expect to find. This will determine the number of test points to be used and the care to be used in evaluating suspected discontinuities.

A discontinuity indication should not be considered as a discontinuity until its origin is determined by making tests at as many angles as possible. This ensures the indication is from a discontinuity and not a result of a reflection from an irregular shape in the specimen or due to a change in metallurgical structure.

If the initial test is made using a straight beam, a discontinuity indication should be examined from various angles using angle beam techniques. In many cases, where irregularly-shaped specimens are being examined, the beam should be plotted on a drawing of the specimen to determine the angle to be chosen for an angle beam test.

Suppose that the back surface of a test specimen lies at an angle of 20° to the front surface. What will be the effect on a normal A-scan display considering that the basic elements of the display always include front and back surface indications under normal conditions?

No effect . . . . **Page 2-29**
Loss of back surface reflection . . . . **Page 2-32**

That is right. If the back surface lies at an angle of 20° relative to the front surface there will be a loss of back surface reflection, since the sound beam will be reflected from the angled surface at an angle of 40° to the examination surface within the test specimen. If you'd like, review the illustration on page 2-29.

With most pulse-echo/through-transmission test instruments, you can control the length of the ultrasonic pulse generated by the test instrument. In addition, by adjusting pulse length, you can control the width of the initial pulse which can mask near surface discontinuities. The illustration below shows how the pulse length will affect the ability of the test instrument to locate discontinuities near the surface.

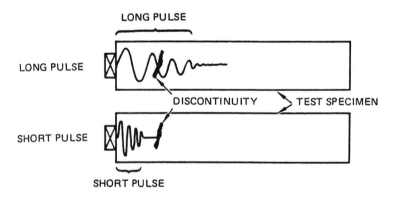

A long pulse blocks the receiver during the period of transmission of sound and covers up reflections from the discontinuity. When the pulse length is shortened, the receiver is not blocked when the reflection returns, but less energy is transmitted into the test specimen.

Should the test instrument be adjusted for a long or a short pulse when testing a thick specimen with a suspected discontinuity about 10 inches (254 mm) below the surface?

Long pulse . . . . **Page 2-34**
Short Pulse . . . . **Page 2-37**

Correct. Only longitudinal waves are introduced into the test specimen. The beam is being transmitted into the specimen at right angles to the test surface and there is no refraction at the interface to cause the mode conversion that produces shear waves.

In angle beam testing, the sound beam is transmitted into the test specimen at an angle to the test surface. To accomplish this, the transducer is placed behind a wedge of material, usually Lucite (or plexiglass) so that the sound will be introduced into the test material at an angle.

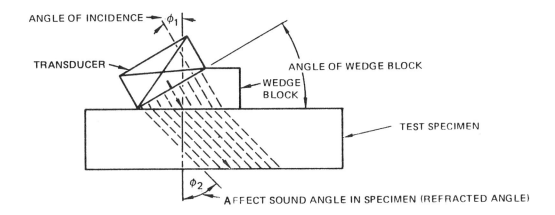

The angle of incidence of the sound beam at the surface of the test specimen is determined by the fixed angle of the plexiglass wedge.

Which of the following characteristics determines the angle of the sound beam in the test specimen?

Acoustic impedance .... **Page 2-35**
Velocity of sound .... **Page 2-38**

Correct. Any time you are checking for discontinuities that are suspected to lie several inches (centimeters) from the test surface, a longer pulse will give better penetrating power.

Let's now discuss the techniques used in transmitting ultrasound into a test specimen.

First, what is straight beam testing? As the name implies, the ultrasonic beam is caused to enter the test specimen at a 90° angle to the test surface by placing the transducer face in a plane parallel to the test surface. The following illustration shows transmission of a signal into a test specimen, reflection from a discontinuity, and the resulting A-scan display.

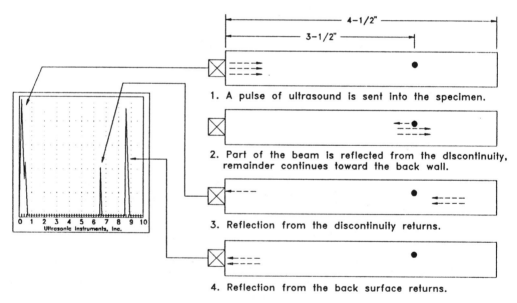

1. A pulse of ultrasound is sent into the specimen.

2. Part of the beam is reflected from the discontinuity, remainder continues toward the back wall.

3. Reflection from the discontinuity returns.

4. Reflection from the back surface returns.

In the above illustration are the waves produced longitudinal waves or shear waves?

Longitudinal waves . . . . **Page 2-33**
Shear waves . . . . **Page 2-36**

Your selection is incorrect.   "Acoustic impedance" is the product of
longitudinal wave velocity in the material and its density. The angle of the
sound beam in the test specimen is determined by the *velocity of sound*
in that *particular material* as compared to the *velocity of sound* in the
plexiglass wedge.

Turn ahead to page 2-38.

It looks like you have forgotten the difference between longitudinal and shear waves. In longitudinal waves, the particle motion is in the direction of sound wave travel. That is the type of wave produced in a test specimen when the sound beam is directed at right angles to the test surface. Shear waves are normally produced only by refraction when the sound beam travels at an angle from a medium of one velocity to a medium of a different velocity.

Turn back to page 2-33.

Your selection was not the correct one. A depth of 10 inches (254 mm) can be considered to be relatively deep for ultrasonic testing and the pulse length should be adjusted to give the best penetrating power at that sound-path distance.

A short pulse provides that only a few cycles of sound energy will be transmitted by the transducer. There is less ultrasonic power in this shorter pulse than in one where there are more cycles of energy transmitted by the transducer. Therefore, to test at a depth of 10 inches (254 mm), the test instrument should be adjusted to give a long pulse.

Turn back to page 2-34.

Correct. You remembered that the angle of the sound beam in a test specimen is determined by the relationship of the velocity of sound in the test specimen and the velocity of sound in the plexiglass wedge—Snell's Law.

You will recall that a refracted longitudinal wave and a shear wave component will be produced by mode conversion when the angle of incidence of the entering sound beam is other than 0° or perpendicular to the surface. As the incident angle increases, refraction of the longitudinal wave increases until there comes a point where total reflection of this wave occurs (refraction exceeds 90°) and all that is left in the test specimen is a shear wave. You will recall that this angle is the first critical angle.

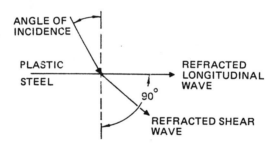

Turn to the next page.

In practice, the angle of the sound beam in the test specimen is usually the critical factor. Based on the velocity of sound in the wedge and in the test specimen, a wedge should be selected that will produce the angle required by the test procedure. Either shear or longitudinal waves, or both, can exist in the test specimen, so the actual type desired must be known. With the following known factors, it is easy to calculate the required wedge angle.

- The desired angle in the test specimen
- The velocity in the wedge
- The velocity in the material

Will the angle of refraction in the test specimen be greater or less as the relative velocities in the wedge and test specimen become more nearly equal?

Greater .... **Page 2-40**

Less .... **Page 2-42**

Your answer is not correct. Let's see if we can clarify the picture a bit.

Consider the path that the sonic beam follows through the two materials. Refraction causes the beam path to be bent as shown here.

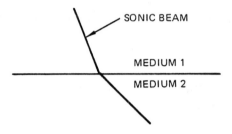

Now, the greater the difference in the sonic velocity of the two materials, the more the beam is bent.

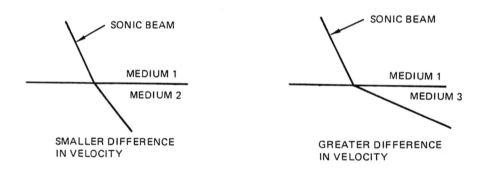

In the view on the left above, the ultrasonic velocity in medium 2 is close to the ultrasonic velocity in medium 1. In the view on the right, the ultrasonic velocity in medium 3 is much greater than the ultrasonic velocity in medium 1.

Now can you see that as the relative velocities in the wedge and test specimen become more nearly equal the angle of refraction becomes smaller?

Turn ahead to page 2-42.

When choosing a wedge, it is most often desirable to avoid those angles that produce both longitudinal and shear waves at the same time and at similar intensities.   Without question, the interpretation of the data becomes more difficult when two waves are traveling through the test specimen at different velocities and at different angles.

The problem of trying to determine which wave is providing a reflection from a particular discontinuity can be solved by operators familiar with such interpretations.

Turn ahead to page 2-43.

That's right. The angle of refraction becomes less as the relative velocities of sound in the wedge and test specimen become more nearly equal. This is shown by rearrangement of the basic Snell's Law formula as follows:

$$\sin \phi_2 = \frac{V_2 \sin \phi_1}{V_1}$$

The angle of refraction is directly proportional to the ratio of velocity of ultrasound in the test specimen to the velocity in the wedge. As this ratio approaches 1, the sines of the two angles, and therefore the size of the angles, become more nearly equal.

The following table lists the velocity of ultrasound and the resultant wavelength of longitudinal waves in some of the more common materials.

MATERIAL	VELOCITY IN PER S	WAVELENGTH AT FREQUENCIES INDICATED		
		1 MHz	2-1/4 MHz	5 MHz
ALUMINUM	245,000	.245 IN.	.109 IN.	.049 IN.
STEEL	229,000	.229	.102	.046
NICKEL	219,000	.219	.097	.044
MAGNESIUM	210,000	.210	.093	.042
COPPER	182,000	.182	.081	.036
BRASS	174,000	.174	.077	.035
LEAD	84,000	.084	.037	.017
GLASS	205,000	.205	.091	.041
LUCITE	105,000	.105	.047	.021
WATER	57,000	.057	.025	.011
AIR	13,900	.014	.006	.003

Assuming a constant Lucite wedge angle of 30°, use the above table and your knowledge of Snell's Law to determine if copper or aluminum will provide the greatest angle of refraction.

Copper .... **Page 2-44**

Aluminum .... **Page 2-46**

The illustrations below depict two different examinations. View A is of a routine shear wave examination and shows a calibration reflector, but no discontinuity. View B is of a *bimodal* examination, that is, an examination utilizing both shear *and* longitudinal wave modes. We can clearly see several indications on the CRT in this view; however, the same calibration reflector was used. Let's not dwell on exactly what caused these indications at this point, but you can see what complications such examinations might bring about!

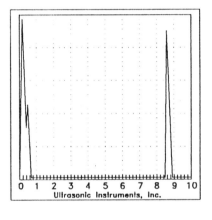

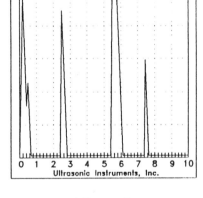

View A   View B

Let's look at a practical example of the problems you might encounter considering we've not yet mastered such screen interpretations.

Turn ahead to page 2-47.

Did you guess on this one? You either guessed or you failed to substitute the proper values in the equation. We aren't interested in the size of the angle of refraction, therefore you do not need to refer to a trigonometry table.   All that is needed here is to refer to the table and obtain the constants that will give the ratio of velocities between the two mediums.

The velocity in Lucite is 105,000 inches (2.67 km) per second which remains constant. The velocity of ultrasound in copper is 182,000 inches (4.62 km) per second, and in aluminum 245,000 inches (6.45 km) per second. Substituting these values in the equation gives the following results:

$$\sin \phi \ (copper) = \frac{V \ (copper) \ X \ \sin \phi \ (Lucite)}{V \ (Lucite)}$$

$$= \frac{182,000 \ X \ \sin \phi \ (Lucite)}{105,000}$$

$$= 1.73 \ X \ \sin \phi \ (Lucite)$$

and:

$$\sin \phi \ (aluminum) = \frac{V \ (aluminum) \ X \ \sin \phi \ (Lucite)}{V \ (Lucite)}$$

$$= \frac{245,000 \ X \ \sin \phi \ (Lucite)}{105,000}$$

$$= 2.33 \ X \ \sin \phi \ (Lucite)$$

Turn to the next page.

You will recall that as the wedge incident angle is increased to the point that the shear wave refracted angle is equal to 90°, we have what is known as the *second critical angle* and no shear wave energy enters the test specimen. A component of sound energy still exists parallel to the interface, however, and this component of energy is known as "surface waves" or "Rayleigh waves."

Refer back to the chart on page 2-46 (or 2-50). Which of the following wedge angles will produce surface waves of the greatest amplitude in steel?

63° . . . . **Page 2-51**
65° . . . . **Page 2-54**

Your selection is incorrect which indicates you did not read the chart correctly. Here's the chart again.

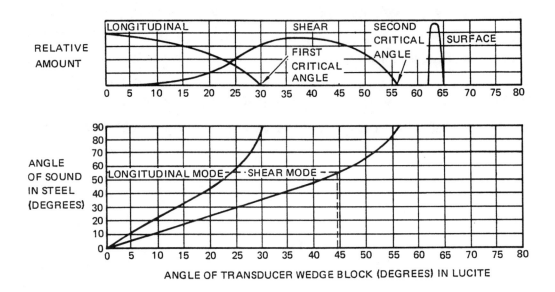

Read across the bottom of the lower chart to where a 45° wedge angle is indicated as stated in the question. Now read up until you come to the shear mode curve. Read across to the vertical line at the left where the angles in the test specimen are indicated. This is shown to be between 50° and 60° or very nearly 57° rather than 63° as you selected.

Turn back to page 2-48.

Very good. A wedge angle of 63° will produce surface waves of greater amplitude in steel than will a wedge angle of 65°.

A surface wave penetrates the test surface to a depth of only about one wavelength and is therefore only adaptable for detection of surface or near surface discontinuities. Since the wave travels on the surface, it will be damped by a liquid so it is only adaptable for contact testing.

A unique feature of surface waves is that they will follow the contour of a test specimen around radii, fillets, and other irregular features (as shown in the following illustration) provided the radius of the contours are large in comparison to the wavelength of the sound wave.

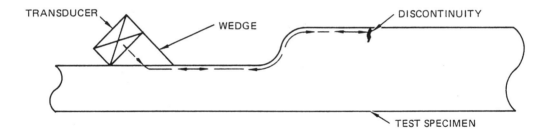

Typical applications for the use of surface waves are:

● Inspection of surfaces of test specimens for cracks caused by fatigue, heat treating, etc.
● Detection of tool marks or other stress risers not visible to the eye

Suppose you are testing a specimen with a test surface having a 90° angle. What effect will the angle have on the surface wave?

No effect . . . . **Page 2-52**
Reflection of the surface wave . . . . **Page 2-55**

Your answer is not correct. A surface wave will go around a contour whose radius is long with respect to one wavelength, but a 90° angle effectively has no radius. The result will be reflection of the sound wave.

The thing to keep in mind is that it's the *radius* around a turn that makes the difference in whether a wave follows a contour or whether it is reflected. If the ultrasonic operator interprets the reasons for a reflection incorrectly, one could assume that the indication of the 90° angle on the CRT shows a crack on the test surface or immediately beneath the surface.

Turn ahead to page 2-55.

The same general rules that are used for other wave modes are used in interpretation of reflections when using plate waves. Sound is transmitted into the test specimen by a transducer and is reflected by a discontinuity or corner of the specimen. The reflection appears in the normal manner.

The choice of a particular plate wave is not critical. The main problem in using plate waves is to cause the energy to propagate through the specimen and reflect back from a discontinuity. In many practical cases, a transducer that is designed to produce shear or surface waves in a larger or heavier test specimen will produce plate waves in relatively thin materials.

Plate waves are extremely useful in the detection of laminations in thin materials. To the wave, the lamination appears as a change in thickness and a portion will be reflected back for display on the CRT. Another application is the detection of a lack of bond in thin laminar constructions (or composites), such as multiple sheets that are cemented or brazed together.

Is the following statement true or false? The propagation of plate (Lamb) waves is NOT dependent on the material properties of the test specimen.

True . . . . **Page 2-56**

False . . . . **Page 2-58**

It looks as if you guessed on this one. Reference to the chart below indicates the maximum amplitude of surface waves occurs at wedge angles between 63° and 64°. In this case your selection should have been 63° for a practical value.

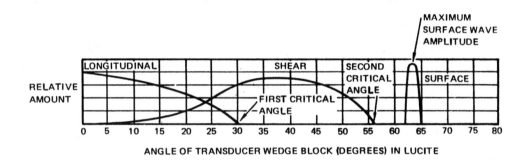

ANGLE OF TRANSDUCER WEDGE BLOCK (DEGREES) IN LUCITE

Look at the chart again to see the relationship of the point where the shear mode ceases to exist and the surface wave mode is effective in relation to the angle of the wedge.

Turn back to page 2-51.

That's right. A 90° angle on a test surface will cause the reflection of a surface wave, since this angle has no radius.

When the material to be tested is very thin (one surface wavelength or less) a special type of wave mode can exist in the sheet. You will recall this is a "plate wave" or "Lamb wave" that is produced by angular incidence of the sound beam and mode conversion at the interface.

Plate waves do not have a single velocity in one material as do the other wave modes. There is a whole family of plate waves of which any one or combinations of more than one may exist simultaneously, depending on the five factors of: (1) frequency, (2) thickness of the sheet, (3) sound velocity in the wedge, (4) incident angle of the wedge, and (5) type of material. The relationship of these factors is shown in the following illustration. It can be seen that by changing one or more of these factors, it is possible to produce conditions where plate waves of various velocities will or will not propagate.

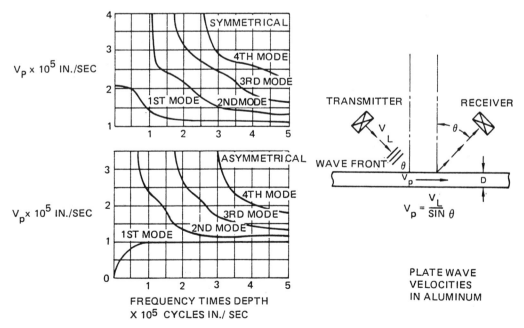

Turn back to page 2-53.

You seem to have forgotten the factors that determine the existence of plate waves. Plate waves are dependent on five factors: (1) frequency, (2) thickness of test specimen, (3) velocity of sound in the wedge, (4) incident angle of the wedge, and (5) type of material.

Since items (2) and (5) pertain only to the material, it follows that the propagation of plate waves is at least partially dependent on the properties of the material in the test specimen.

Turn ahead to page 2-58.

Transducer combinations in two-transducer testing systems may be classified into two groups as follows:

- The most common combines transmit-receive search units with two transducers mounted in a single housing and acoustically insulated from each other. Each transducer is connected separately to the transmitter and receiver-amplifier units. This combination is illustrated in View A below. We referred to this earlier in another Volume as a dual-element probe.
- Separate transmitting and receiving transducers with separate electrical connections to the transmitter and receiver-amplifier units. This principle is illustrated in View B.

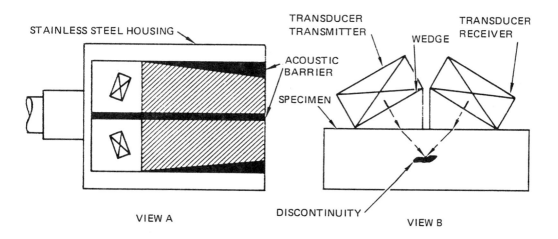

Turn ahead to page 2-59.

Correct. The propagation of plate (Lamb) waves is dependent on the material properties of the test specimen, among other factors. These include frequency, thickness of the specimen, angle of incidence of the wedge, and sound velocity in the wedge.

Let's now consider the use of two transducers in contact testing. Throughout these first chapters there have been references to the use of two transducers principally in the discussions of through-transmission testing. Although not extensively used in practical testing applications, there are situations where two transducers will provide more satisfactory test results in certain applications of *pulse-echo* testing.

You learned that the through-transmission system operates on the principle of transmitting sound waves through a test specimen with one transducer and receiving on a second transducer. A discontinuity is indicated by a reduction in the magnitude of sound energy available at the receiving transducer. In two-transducer pulse-echo testing, sound waves are transmitted by a transmitting transducer and discontinuity *reflections* are picked up at a receiving transducer.

Turn back to page 2-57.

The principle of two-transducer pulse-echo testing is illustrated below with a typical view of the indication received on the CRT. A single transducer used for both transmitting and receiving cannot detect discontinuities until its function as a transmitter is complete, which results in a zone near the surface that the test system cannot "see." A two-transducer system can detect discontinuities before the transmission of the pulse is complete, since the receiving probe is always "listening."

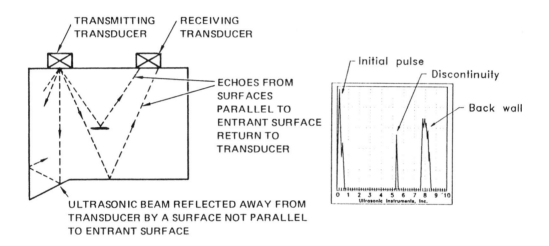

Would you say that a two-transducer pulse-echo system is more sensitive to the detection of *all* discontinuities than a single transducer system.

Yes .... Page 2-60

No .... Page 2-61

You're wrong. A two-transducer pulse-echo system is more sensitive to the detection of discontinuities *close to the surface* of the test specimen. But sensitivity to the near surface discontinuities is the only area where the two-transducer pulse-echo system is the more sensitive.

For all practical purposes, sensitivity to discontinuities is the same for both single- and two-transducer pulse-echo testing in that portion of the test specimen between the areas normally occupied by the front and back surface reflections.

Turn to the next page.

That's right. A two-transducer pulse-echo system is *not* more sensitive to the detection of *all* discontinuities. It is more sensitive only in detecting discontinuities *very near to the surface.* Sensitivity is about the same in the area of the specimen between the normal location of the front and back surface reflections.

Before proceeding to the application of contact testing to the various materials and the manufacturing processes that may be inspected, let's first review the more important points you have learned in this chapter.

Turn to the next page.

CHAPTER REVIEW

_____ 1. The selection of ultrasonic test equipment for contact testing depends largely on the test _____ and test _____.

    A.   situation, procedure
    B.   operator, day
    C.   operator, specimen
    D.   day, time

_____ 2. The greatest limitation of contact testing is the difficulty in maintaining uniform acoustical _____ between the transducer and test specimen.

    A.   segregation
    B.   attenuation
    C.   reflection
    D.   coupling

_____ 3. The substance that must be placed between the transducer and test surface during contact testing is called a:

    A.   gel.
    B.   segregate.
    C.   absorber.
    D.   couplant.

4. A test specimen with a coarse-grained internal structure will require selection of a _____ frequency for testing.

A. high
B. low

5. When testing a specimen that has a rough surface, a _____ oil should be used as a couplant.

A. thin
B. heavy
C. light
D. clear

6. A rough test surface may cause the sound beam to _____ when testing.

A. revert
B. focus
C. converge
D. scatter

7. At a given ultrasonic test frequency, a _____ transducer will produce the least beam spread.

A. large
B. small
C. round
D. square

_____ 8. Assume that a test is being made on a 10-foot-long (3 meter) specimen. The _____ transducer would be selected to give the best penetrating power at the test frequency of 2.25 MHz.

A. 0.1 inch (2.5 mm)
B. 0.25 inch (6.3 mm)
C. 0.5 inch (12.7 mm)
D. 1 inch (25.4 mm)

_____ 9. In ultrasonic test instruments, the pulse length is variable. When a test is to be conducted on a thick specimen, a _____ pulse will give the best results.

A. shorter
B. taller
C. longer
D. thinner

_____ 10. Plastic wedges are used for obtaining a specific refracted angle of testing in _____ testing.

A. straight beam
B. immersion
C. angle beam
D. through-contact

_____ 11. The ability of an ultrasonic testing system to detect discontinuities depends on pulse length and frequency, among other factors. A combination of _____ pulse length and _____ frequency will give the best discontinuity detection.

A. short, high
B. short, low
C. long, high
D. long, low

_____ 12. A test is to be made on a rough vertical surface. With a choice to be made between engine oil and water with a wetting agent as couplant, _____ is the best selection.

A. water
B. engine oil

_____ 13. Any mode of wave propagation can be produced when using a variable angle:

A. couplant.
B. cable.
C. pulser.
D. transducer.

14. In straight beam testing, the wave mode is:

A. shear.
B. surface.
C. plate.
D. longitudinal.

15. In angle beam testing, the angle of incidence at the surface of the test specimen is determined by the angle of the Lucite wedge. The _____ of sound in the test specimen is another factor that helps to determine the angle that the sound will travel in the specimen.

A. velocity
B. color
C. intensity
D. wavelength

16. Both shear and longitudinal wave components are present to a significant degree when using certain angles for angle beam testing. For practical applications, the _____ wave should be eliminated.

A. shear
B. longitudinal
C. surface
D. plate

_____   17.   When the angle of refraction of the shear waves is equal to 90°, surface waves are produced. A unique feature of surface waves is that they will follow the contour of a test specimen provided the radius of the contour is large in comparison to the _____ of the wave.

A.   frequency
B.   amplitude
C.   wavelength
D.   rotation

_____   18.   Plate (Lamb) waves, which can be produced in very _____ materials, are extremely useful in detecting the presence of _____.

A.   heavy, discontinuities
B.   thick, cracks
C.   thin, laminations
D.   light, voids

Turn to the next page for answers to these review questions.

ANSWERS TO REVIEW QUESTIONS
FOR CHAPTER 2

Question & Answer		Reference Page(s)
1.	A	2-3, 2-5
2.	D	2-1, 2-23
3.	D	2-23
4.	B	2-14
5.	B	2-23, 2-26
6.	D	2-3
7.	A	2-18
8.	D	2-20, 2-24
9.	C	2-34
10.	C	2-33
11.	A	2-17
12.	B	2-26, 2-28
13.	D	2-33
14.	D	2-33, 2-34
15.	A	2-42
16.	B	2-47
17.	C	2-51
18.	C	2-53

Turn to the next page and begin Chapter 3.

CHAPTER 3

APPLICATION OF CONTACT TESTING

Now let's consider the application of contact testing to materials of varying shapes, sizes, composition, and internal structure. The first application that we will discuss is the testing of castings.

The lower range of test frequencies is generally used to test castings due to their coarse-grained internal structure. Many of the *very* coarse-grained castings are not easily tested ultrasonically due to the extreme scattering of the sound beam by the grain structure. This also depends on the type of casting process. Examples are alloys of brass, stainless steel, titanium, and cast iron.

In most tests, when the back surface indication is visible, there will be several heavily-damped stray indications between the front surface indication and back surface indication that are due to the internal structure.

If you have a choice between a 1.0-megahertz (MHz) transducer and a 2.25-MHz transducer for testing a casting, which would be the most practical to select?

2.25-MHz transducer . . . . **Page 3-3**
1.0-MHz transducer . . . . **Page 3-5**

Correct. You will be most likely to detect discontinuities in a forging if the inspection is made at several angles to the direction of working. Though the grain of the metal is oriented in the direction of working, forgings may not provide easy access for testing.

The problems of testing bar stock are similar to those encountered in tests of forgings. If an ingot similar to the forging previously discussed is rolled or stretched into a long configuration (i.e., be it round, square, or octagonal) the configuration is now classed as bar stock. Shrinkage, inclusions, or porosity are now changed into seams, laps, centerline piping, or some other form of elongated discontinuities as shown in the following illustration.

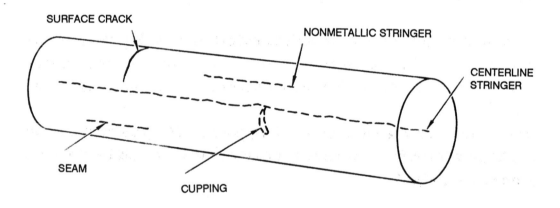

Turn ahead to page 3-7.

The selection of 2.25 MHz in preference to 1.0 MHz for testing a casting is not the best of the two choices available. The large grain structure inherent in most castings dictates that the lower frequency be used to reduce spurious indications from the coarse grains. A frequency of 1.0 MHz will provide better penetrating power and be less sensitive to grain structure variations than 2.25 MHz.

Turn ahead to page 3-5.

Illustrated below is a typical rotating shaft. Note the types and number of scans suggested for complete volumetric coverage of the article.

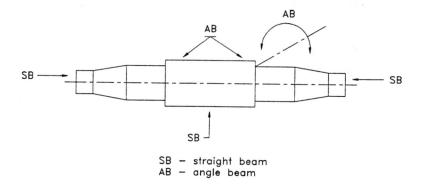

SB — straight beam
AB — angle beam

Discontinuities that may be detected in forgings are nonmetallic inclusions, seams, forging bursts, cracks, and flaking. Typical indications are illustrated below.

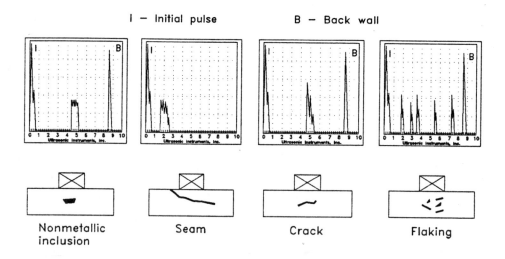

I — Initial pulse   B — Back wall

Nonmetallic inclusion   Seam   Crack   Flaking

From which direction should the inspection be made in order to most likely detect discontinuities in a forging?

From several directions on the forging . . . . **Page 3-2**
Normal to direction of working of the forging . . . . **Page 3-6**

That is correct. The best results will be obtained if a 1.0-MHz transducer is used to test a casting in comparison to those that would be obtained from using a 2.25-MHz transducer.

In contrast to castings, many forgings are of uniform size and shape and are good candidates for ultrasonic testing. This includes hollow, rectangular, and round or multifaceted shapes, such as pump shafts and turbine rotors. These products can be made of many metals and alloys. Testing of forgings is normally accomplished at frequencies of 1.0 to 5.0 MHz with both straight beam and angle beam probes. This is because discontinuities can be at a variety of orientations to the examination surface.

Turn back to page 3-4.

Incorrect. Let's take a look at what is meant by "the direction of working."

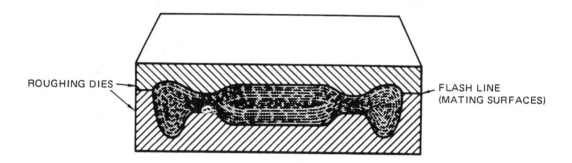

The illustration above shows an article lying in the dies with which it was formed. The illustration also shows, by means of the grain lines in the article, how the metal had to flow in order for the article to be formed. The grain lines lie in, and identify, the direction of working.

Discontinuities which may be present in the parent metal will also be flattened and forced to follow these grain lines, but the shape of the forging indicates that discontinuities could lie in almost any direction. Therefore, it would be best to test the forging at several angles to assure the highest probability of properly orienting the sound beam with the discontinuities.

Turn back to page 3-2.

A bar may be tested from the end so the sound beam is transmitted through its length. If access to both ends is possible, it should be tested from both ends. Testing from both ends allows the use of lower gain settings on the instrument. The use of screen divisions will enable an accurate determination of the locations of discontinuities.

If a good back surface reflection can be obtained by sending the sound beam through the entire length of the bar with no significant discontinuity indications, the bar can be considered free of gross discontinuities. There is not likely to be seriously elongated piping or seams present in the specimen if a strong back surface reflection is obtained.

Will an end-to-end test of a 10-foot (3-meter) bar that results in a large back surface reflection and no large discontinuity indications mean the bar has no discontinuities?

No . . . . **Page 3-8**
Yes . . . . **Page 3-10**

That's right. An end-to-end test that results in a large back surface reflection with no large discontinuity indications does not mean the bar is completely free of discontinuities. There may be discontinuities that are oriented parallel to the length of the bar that are not detected by this approach. Whether or not additional testing is required will depend on the requirements of the test.

Further testing of bar stock can be made by the "diametrical" technique. In this technique, the transducer is applied to the side of the bar so that the sound is transmitted through, and reflected by, the opposite side. Depending on the diameter of the bar, this technique may not be very efficient in transmitting sound into the bar due to insufficient contact surface between the transducer and entry surface. The coupling of sound from the transducer to the entry surface of the bar may be improved by using a wedge that is contoured to the radius of the bar as illustrated.

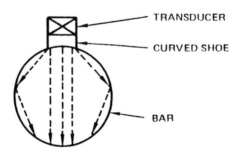

Turn to the next page.

When complete diametrical testing is not practical, the bar may be scanned diametrically approximately 90° apart along the length of the bar. Any elongated piping, seams, or elongated porosity can be easily located using this technique.

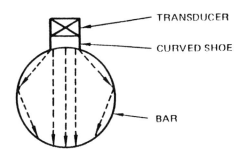

The idealized illustration above shows the sound beam entering the bar as longitudinal waves.

Under actual test conditions, what wave modes will be present in the bar?

Longitudinal waves .... **Page 3-11**
Longitudinal and shear waves .... **Page 3-13**

Your analysis in this case is not correct. End testing resulting in a strong back surface reflection and no large discontinuity indications will indicate merely that there are no large discontinuities. There may be discontinuities oriented parallel to the direction of the sound beam that are not detected. Depending upon the test requirements and the ultimate use of the specimen, the discontinuities that cannot be detected by end testing may be sufficiently large to cause rejection of the specimen if the test is made transverse to the length of the bar.

Turn back to page 3-8.

Don't be fooled by the illustration which shows most of the sound entering straight into the specimen. Actually, the curved surface of the bar will create a varying angle of incidence across the width of the sound beam that will cause refraction to varying degrees. The refracted beams will have both *longitudinal* and *shear* components. That should have been your selection for a correct answer.

Turn ahead to page 3-13.

When the plate is sufficiently thick that the first back surface reflection is distinct from the initial pulse on the CRT, a multiple reflection pattern as shown in View A below may be displayed on the CRT. A reduction in the spacing of the multiple reflection pattern as shown in View B indicates the presence of discontinuities. View A assumes a plate with no discontinuities and the distance between each pulse is the plate thickness. Note that in View B the horizontal distance between pulses is less than in View A due to reflections from a mid-wall lamination.

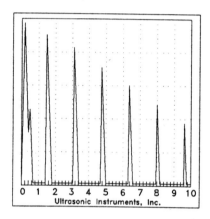

View A
No lamination

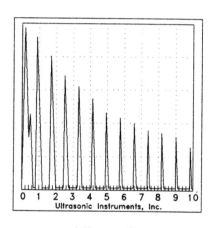

View B
Lamination

If a 100% test is to be made of a sheet of steel 4 feet (1.2 meters) by 8 feet (2.4 meters), would it be more practical to initially perform a detailed or gross straight beam scan?

Detailed scan .... **Page 3-14**
Gross scan .... **Page 3-16**

Excellent. You correctly determined that the curved surface of the bar will cause varying angles of incidence across the width of the sound beam resulting in refraction within the specimen and production of both longitudinal and shear waves.

Rolled sheet and plate materials may be tested with either a straight beam or an angle beam. Straight beam testing has the advantages of being able to pick up signals from laminations readily, discontinuities can be pinpointed, and their extremities can be easily and accurately determined. Straight beam testing, however, cannot be used on a sheet that is too thin to allow the first back surface reflection to clear the initial pulse. Recall that in an earlier Volume, we suggested the use of a plexiglass stand-off to overcome this problem. Another limitation is that straight beam testing is very time consuming if 100% testing is required.

Let's look at straight beam testing of plate.

Return to the previous page.

Your answer is not the best selection. Before going to the trouble of setting up and scanning the plate in detail, it is best to do a gross check to determine if the plate has large discontinuities that are sufficient to cause immediate rejection of the plate. If a large number of sheets are to be tested, considerable time can be saved by following this procedure.

Turn ahead to page 3-16.

That's correct.   Discontinuities in a rolled plate are more likely to be oriented *parallel* to the surface rather than at an angle to the surface.   This is due to the working of the metal which orients the grain structure and discontinuities in the direction of rolling.

Turn ahead to page 3-20.

You're right. Why waste time setting up and scanning a plate with a detail scan if the plate contains large discontinuities that make it obviously unacceptable? Gross discontinuities can be detected rapidly by a sampling of straight beam tests. If these tests are satisfactory, then the operator can proceed with the angle beam test if appropriate.

Turn ahead to page 3-18.

Your selection is not correct. Discontinuities are most likely to be oriented *parallel* to the surface in a rolled plate.

A billet, as poured, has a random grain structure and the discontinuities are scattered in a random fashion. The rolling process will refine the grain structure and align the grain in the direction of rolling. Discontinuities will likewise be aligned in the direction of rolling which will make them parallel to the surface.

Turn back to page 3-15.

For example, let's assume that a plate 4 feet (1.2 meters) by 8 feet (2.4 meters) by 1/2 inch (12.7 mm) is to be tested. The plate should first be divided into a checkerboard-type grid with approximately 6 inches (15.2 cm) between grid lines. (It is not necessary to actually draw grid lines on the plate—imaginary grid lines are sufficient.) The plate should first be spot checked in each of the grid squares with a straight beam transducer. This type of random sampling will give the operator an idea of the amount of laminations present in the plate. If any are found, more detailed examination of the outline of the defective areas can be made at that time. If the grid check doesn't show any gross laminations in the plate, the angle beam transducer can then be used for a more thorough scanning of the entire plate area.

How are discontinuities in a rolled plate likely to be oriented?

Parallel to surface .... **Page 3-15**
At an angle to the surface .... **Page 3-17**

Unless otherwise specified, a calibration notch should be approximately 5% to 10% of the plate thickness. Locate and use the notch for a 1/2-inch-thick (12.7 mm) plate as follows:

- Place the notch approximately 2 inches (50.8 mm) from one end of the reference test plate so that back surface reflections from the edge of the plate will not interfere with interpretation of signals from the reference notch.

- Using a suitable couplant, place the transducer approximately 2 inches (50.8 mm) from the notch and adjust the gain of the instrument so that the signal from the notch is 50% FSH. Move the transducer toward and away from the notch until the indication reaches its greatest amplitude. Adjust the gain so that the indication is 100% FSH.

- Move the transducer back about 1.5 inches (38.1 mm) from this position and note the amplitude of the signal on the CRT. After finding its highest peak as above, mark the height of the signal on the face of the CRT with a grease pencil for future reference.

- Repeat this operation at 3 inches (76.2 mm) and 4.5 inches (114.3 mm) from the notch. Reference marks on the CRT indicate the amplitude of the reflected signal that may be expected from the manufactured notch at any of several different distances from the notch.

Assume you are testing a plate in accordance with an ultrasonic test procedure. Would you normally expect the reference notch dimensions to be prescribed by the procedure?

No . . . . **Page 3-21**
Yes . . . . **Page 3-23**

Service induced discontinuities in plate used in many structural steel applications includes surface connected cracking. These often result from repeated cyclic mechanical stresses on members. These cracks are not often detected in a straight beam scan. However, angle beam testing would readily detect and locate such cracks.

Before using an angle beam transducer for inspection of the plate, it is necessary to calibrate such that the amplitude of the reflected sound from a discontinuity of known size can be used as a reference.

Turn back to page 3-19.

Sorry, you are wrong. The dimensions of the reference notch should be prescribed by the ultrasonic test procedure.

The ultrasonic test operator is expected to be capable of locating discontinuities in a test specimen, compare them with a certain prescribed standard and, from this comparison, make a determination if the specimen should or should not be accepted.

The size of the reference notch and distribution of discontinuities that are acceptable should be available to the operator *in the test procedure*. The use to which a specimen is to be put will, in most cases, determine the size and number of discontinuities that can be tolerated.

Turn ahead to page 3-23.

Illustrated below is the finger damping concept.

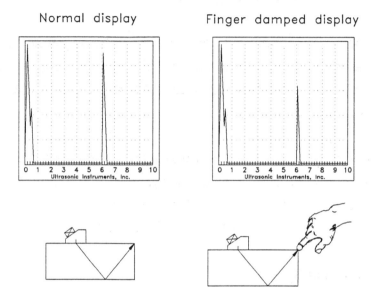

Once the location of the discontinuity is known, it is a simple matter to move the transducer to a point equal to one of the surface distances measured from the reference notch. The amplitude of the signal from the discontinuity can then be compared with the signal from the reference notch.

While performing our plate scan, discontinuities that produce indications that are equal to or greater than the amplitude of reflections from the reference notch should be marked and should be further evaluated by testing at different angles after scanning is complete. It is possible that the signal amplitude may be greater at a different angle.

If you receive a stronger signal at one angle than another, does this mean an error was made during scanning?

Yes .... **Page 3-24**
No .... **Page 3-26**

That is right. You can normally expect that the test procedure for testing the plate will specify the dimensions of the reference notch.

Scan the plate by moving the transducer along each side (face) of the plate with the beam angled so that it is reflected from the upper and lower surfaces. A discontinuity that causes an indication to appear is easy to locate in the plate by either using the divisions in the display to measure the distance or the operator's fingers can be moved along the plate in front of the transducer toward the discontinuity. Movement of the fingers along the plate may cause a small signal on the CRT that will move in the direction of the discontinuity. When the fingers are directly over the discontinuity, the signal will be damped. Placing one's fingers over the location of the sound beam on the surface of the component causes a localized change in acoustic impedance. This results in more localized sound transmittance and less reflectance. Such a technique, referred to as "finger damping," is an effective technique for locating the sound beam in a variety of angle beam applications.

Turn back to page 3-22.

Your selection is not correct. When scanning, the sound beam is subject to skipping certain areas of the material as the sound beam bounces between the top and bottom surfaces in traveling across the plate. There are probably some discontinuities that will not be "seen" by the sound beam at all and others that will not be struck by the beam at such an angle that the reflected sound energy reflects the true size of the discontinuities.

Testing at various angles will determine whether the indication received during the initial scan correctly detected the extent of the discontinuity. There definitely was no error made in scanning; it is just one of the characteristics of angle beam testing that must be understood.

Turn ahead to page 3-26.

Excellent. It is quite possible that you will be able to generate plate waves in a plate even though you do not have a variable-angle transducer available. If you have a variety of fixed-angle transducers and various frequencies available to you, you most likely can experiment until you find a combination that will result in the generation of plate waves. If the selection of fixed angles and frequencies is limited, it is unlikely that these waves can be produced.

Turn ahead to page 3-27.

Right—during initial scanning the sound beam may completely miss some discontinuities and may be only partially reflected by others when the sound beam does not strike them at an angle of 90°. It is because some discontinuities may be missed that scanning should be done from a second side. Because of the second possibility, it is necessary to examine the discontinuity at various angles at the correct distance to determine the extent and seriousness of the discontinuity.

The previous discussion of angle beam testing of plate materials has assumed that discontinuities are located in the interior of the plate at such a depth that they could be detected by the use of shear waves.

Suppose now that you want to determine if there are cracks on the surface or just beneath the surface using surface waves. To generate surface waves you need an angle beam transducer with a wedge angle that lies slightly beyond the second critical angle for generating shear waves in that particular type of specimen. You will use the same scanning techniques and use the reference notch in the same manner as you did for shear waves.

In surface wave testing it is extremely important that the surface of the test specimen be free of dirt, oil, and any excess couplant. You will recall that any of these foreign elements will readily attenuate surface waves and the test sensitivity and validity will be reduced.

Assume that you have the task of testing a rolled plate for surface discontinuities. Which surface should you test from?

Either the top or bottom . . . . **Page 3-28**
The top and bottom . . . . **Page 3-30**

Discontinuities in extrusions usually extend lengthwise in the specimen because of elongation in the direction of extrusion. Straight beam techniques and interpretation of discontinuity indications for solid specimens of extrusions are the same as those given for bar stock. Where hollow extrusions are to be tested, it may be more practical to use surface wave techniques as illustrated below.

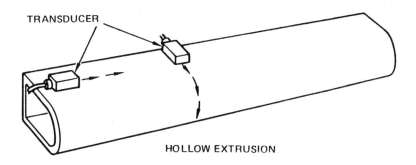

TRANSDUCER

HOLLOW EXTRUSION

The sample shown is curved. It is possible with such a shape to get complete coverage of the specimen by scanning lengthwise and then scanning transversely. The surface waves will follow the curvature of the specimen and be reflected by the sharp edge on the opposite side. Of course this technique will only detect surface discontinuities.

Suppose the extrusion shown in the illustration is aluminum and you do not have an angle beam transducer that will allow you to produce surface waves in the specimen. You do have available an angle beam transducer that will allow you to produce shear waves.

Can the same scanning techniques be used for shear waves as those shown for surface waves?

No . . . . **Page 3-29**
Yes . . . . **Page 3-31**

Have you forgotten the characteristics of surface waves? These waves travel only on the surface and below the surface to a depth of about one wavelength. This isn't very deep when you consider that one wavelength at 5 MHz is 0.002 inch (0.05 mm) in both steel and aluminum.

It will be necessary to scan *both* of the plate surfaces to detect all surface discontinuities. Surface discontinuities are just as bad when they occur on the bottom as when they occur on the top of the plate.

Turn ahead to page 3-30.

Very good. You can't use the same scanning technique for shear waves that you used for surface waves since shear waves will not touch at all points along the surface. The specimen can be tested using shear waves but it will be necessary to do additional scanning to obtain complete coverage of both the upper and lower surfaces of this hollow specimen.

Consider now the techniques to be used in testing pipe and tubing by ultrasonic means. The illustration below shows what happens to a sound beam that strikes the surface at an angle other than perpendicular. The refracted sound beam is transmitted around the wall of the tubular specimen.

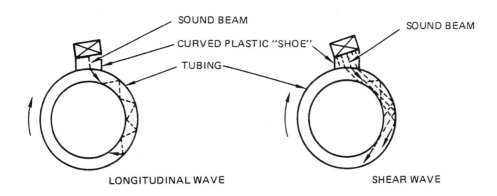

Sound propagates around the wall in a zigzag pattern as either longitudinal or shear waves. Due to the undesirable existence of both shear and longitudinal waves when testing at less than first critical angle, most testing on specimens of tubular shape is accomplished with shear waves between the first and second critical angles.

What type of transducer would you select to conduct an ultrasonic test on a section of pipe with an outside diameter of 6 inches (152.4 mm)?

Straight beam . . . . **Page 3-33**
Curved shoe, angle beam . . . . **Page 3-35**

Correct. Of course you have to test both surfaces. Surface waves penetrate only to a depth of about one wavelength. Scanning one surface will only tell you if there are any surface discontinuities on that one side. Then you have to turn the plate over and test the other side using the same techniques.

There is one more technique that you may have to use when you are testing very thin materials using an angle beam—the "plate wave" technique. In materials with a thickness approximately equal to one-half wavelength of the surface wave sound beam, it is not possible to generate shear or surface waves. However, plate waves can be produced in these thin materials if any ultrasonic transmission is possible at all.

It is often difficult to generate plate waves with fixed-angle transducers; therefore, it is desirable to use a variable-angle transducer so the angle can be adjusted to generate plate waves in the test plate.

To generate plate waves using a variable-angle transducer, you place the transducer on the test specimen with suitable couplant and adjust the incident angle of the sound beam to the point that reflections are observed in the display. Then you scan the plate with the transducer set at this angle. Changing the angle of the transducer will result in loss of indications, indicating that plate waves are no longer being produced.

Suppose you do not have a variable-angle transducer available. You do have several fixed-angle transducers at various frequencies. Do you think it is still possible to generate plate waves in the test plate?

Yes . . . . **Page 3-25**
No . . . . **Page 3-32**

Sorry, the scanning technique for shear waves is never the same as that for surface waves. You must remember that a surface wave takes in *all* of the surface that lies in the beam while a shear wave skips some of the surface. For this reason, the scanning technique used with shear waves is more complex than the scanning technique used with surface waves.

Turn back to page 3-29.

Your answer is not the best selection. It was stated that you have available a number of fixed-angle transducers at various frequencies. The thickness of the plate is a fixed quantity as is the velocity of sound in the wedge. However, two of the variables that are a determining factor in generation of plate waves can be adjusted. It will be necessary to experiment by selecting different angles and frequencies and observing the display for an indication that sound waves are being generated. Your answer to the question should have been "yes," although in practical application the range of angles and transducer frequencies available to you may not give the correct combination for generation of plate waves.

Turn back to page 3-25.

Your answer isn't the best one. A straight beam transducer will not produce a wave that will travel around the wall of the pipe. The main portion of the beam will enter the test surface perpendicularly, travel to the opposite wall and reflect back to the transducer, providing an ultrasonic test of only a small area of the pipe's circumference. It will be more practical to use an angle beam transducer which will cause the sound to enter the specimen at an angle and travel around the tube.

Turn ahead to page 3-35.

Suppose that a notch is cut in the pipe directly opposite the position of the transducer as illustrated. The reflection from this notch appears at the 6th screen division on the CRT. Because we are examining the pipe circumferentially, the precise location of the discontinuities will be a bit more involved. We won't tackle that issue here.

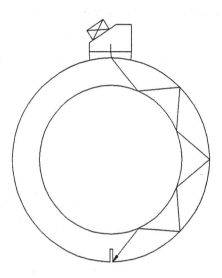
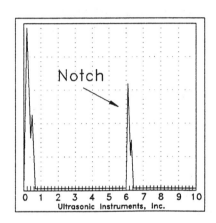

Assume that a shear wave is being transmitted into a pipe in a clockwise direction. A discontinuity exists at a point 220° around the circumference from the point of entry of the sound beam. Will this discontinuity indication appear to the left or right of the indication directly opposite the probe?

Left . . . . **Page 3-36**
Right . . . . **Page 3-38**

Right—an angle beam transducer will project sound into the pipe wall at an angle and the sound beam will travel around the circumference of the pipe in a zigzag manner.

There are certain limitations to the use of contact testing for testing pipe and tubing, although this technique may be used to transmit shear waves around the circumference of pipe as small as 1-3/4 inch (44.5 mm) outside diameter. There are lower limitations to the diameter of pipe that can be tested by this technique but no practical limits for large diameter pipes.

In addition to the size limitations, there are serious limitations to the speed with which the length of a specimen can be scanned manually using a contoured contact wedge.

If you are selecting a material for the construction of a contact contoured wedge for use in testing a pipe, which of the following materials will you select?

Same as the pipe **3-37**
Same as the typical wedge **3-39**

Sorry. You missed on this one. The distance the beam travels for a 180° discontinuity reveals an indication at the 6th major screen division. If a discontinuity exists at 220° with respect to the transducer, the sound will travel further to reach the discontinuity. The indication will therefore be to the *right* of the indication directly opposing (180°) the search unit.

Turn ahead to page 3-38.

It won't work. Think now what will happen if you try to use a contoured wedge that is the same material as the pipe.

You will get a false surface indication when the sound beam travels from the probe into the contoured wedge.   Results will be anything but satisfactory. You also will receive a reflection from the interface between the contoured wedge and pipe surface - not a complete reflection due to the presence of a good couplant (supposedly). But, with all these spurious reflections, it will be difficult to differentiate these reflections from discontinuities.   Use the same material as the wedge and avoid these difficulties.

Turn ahead to page 3-39.

Excellent. Because the sound travels more than 180° around the pipe, the indication is to the right of the 180° indication.   Indications from discontinuities that exist less than 180° from the transducer will appear to its left. Illustrated below are a couple of examples.

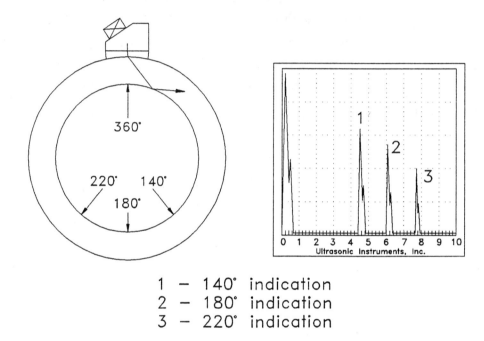

1 — 140° indication
2 — 180° indication
3 — 220° indication

You must remember that the sonic beam continues to travel around the pipe until it is completely attenuated. There is no "end" to the sound path.

Turn ahead to page 3-40.

Correct. The contoured wedge should be made of the same material as the typical wedge, which is normally plexiglass.

Assume now a practical application of testing a steel pipe 6 inches (152.4 mm) in diameter with a 3/4-inch (19 mm) wall. Use of the contact technique utilizing shear wave techniques is assumed with a test frequency of 2.25 MHz. Very little cleaning of the outside surface of the pipe is necessary. The main requirement is that it be free of loose material. Once cleaned, apply some couplant in the scan area.

A 45° angle beam transducer with a Lucite wedge cut to fit the contour of the pipe is used to propagate shear waves which are directed around the circumference of the pipe as illustrated below. The shear waves bounce off the outer and inner surfaces of the pipe wall as they travel around the circumference. The waves travel completely around the pipe and provide no indications on the CRT when there are no discontinuities present.

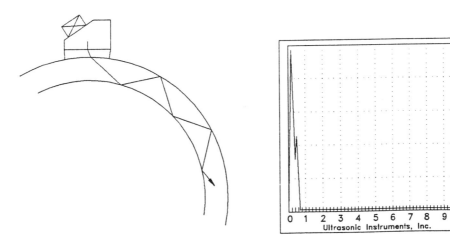

Circumferential scanning of "clean" pipe

Turn back to page 3-34.

Calibration standards for pipe and tubing are often not available as a commercial item; therefore, it is necessary to prepare a standard for comparison with the actual test specimen. This standard usually consists of reference notches, machined into a sample of the test specimen having the same ultrasonic characteristics. A notch is cut in both the inside and outside diameters of the pipe or tube. Unless otherwise specified, each notch should be approximately *1-1/2 inches (38.1 mm) long* and have a depth that approximates *5% to 10% of the wall thickness*.

The transducer is placed on the reference specimen at 90°, 180°, and 270° and reflections obtained from each of the artificial discontinuities. You can then mark the amplitude of the discontinuity indication at each position on the face of the display, possibly with a grease pencil. Electronic DAC circuits can also be utilized to establish a reference amplitude or level.

During testing, discontinuity indication amplitude is compared with the amplitude received from the artificial discontinuities at the indicated distance around the circumference of the specimen.

Is the following statement true or false? The inner and outer calibration notches in a sample piece of pipe should be cut at the same location on the circumference of a thin (less than 1/4-inch-thick [6.3 mm]) pipe.

True . . . . **Page 3-42**
False . . . . **Page 3-44**

Welds may be ultrasonically tested by either straight beam or angle beam techniques, although the angle beam technique is in much wider use.

Straight beam testing of welds is more readily accomplished if the surface of the weld is ground flush (as shown in View A below), while the weld bead may extend above the surfaces joined by the weld when angle beam techniques are used (as shown in View B).

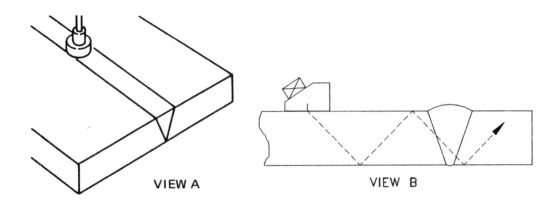

VIEW A   VIEW B

The couplant used in testing welds may be either oil, water with a wetting agent added, or any commercially available ultrasonic couplant. Of course, if the test surface is not smooth it will be necessary to use a more viscous couplant.

When testing a weld with the angle beam technique, do you think you might receive any reflections from the weld area even if there are no discontinuities present?

No .... **Page 3-43**
Yes .... **Page 3-45**

What sort of artificial discontinuity reference would you receive under these conditions? How can you determine if your indication is from the inner or outer surface notch? You can't. You are likely to receive an indication that is a combination of the reflections from each of the notches. It is preferable to place one notch at each end of a reference sample. If for some reason it is necessary to place both notches at the same end of a reference sample, separate them so that they are individually detectable.

Turn ahead to page 3-44.

Well. . . , you *may* receive a reflection from the weld area even if there are no discontinuities present. This most often occurs when there are different materials welded together and there are different alloys used in the weldment. Remember, there is a fusion zone on each side of the weld where it joins the (possibly different) base metal. These fusion zones may cause reflections.

The weld contains metal with a grain structure which is randomly-oriented as compared with the uniform grain structure of the base material joined together. The weld itself is essentially a cast material embedded in a mold created by the base metal forming the joint.

Turn ahead to page 3-45.

That's right. The reference notches on the inner and outer diameters of the reference sample should not be cut at the same location on the circumference of the pipe. They need to be separated so that separate and distinct artificial discontinuity indications can be received for reference purposes. It is preferable that the inner and outer diameter reference notches be placed at opposite ends of a reference sample. If it is necessary that the two notches be placed on the same end of a sample, they should be separated so that they are individually detectable.

Let's proceed now to the consideration of locating discontinuities in welds by means of contact pulse-echo testing.

Welds may contain discontinuities of varying types such as porosity, cracks, lack of fusion, incomplete penetration, and nonmetallic inclusions. The acceptable quality of a weld is an inverse function of the total quantity, shape, and size of discontinuities in some linear distance of the weld. Acceptability also depends on the thickness and properties of the material being welded.

Welds are usually inspected using a test frequency of 1.5, 2.25, or 5 MHz, depending on the nature of the weld discontinuities anticipated, the material joined by the welding process, and the weld filler material.

Turn back to page 3-41.

You certainly might. This most often occurs when there are different materials (carbon steel and stainless steel for example) welded together and there are different alloys used in the weldment. The weld itself is essentially a cast material embedded in a mold created by the base metal forming the joint. Therefore, the fusion zones between the base metal being joined and the weld area may cause indications due to reflections of the ultrasound. Depending on the material being joined and the weld filler material, such reflectors may be more pronounced or not present at all. These are termed "metallurgical" reflectors and most test procedures allow us to ignore them.

Illustrated below are some typical indications of welds *with* metallurgical reflectors. In View A, a satisfactory weld area is shown with the fusion zones clearly indicated. View B shows the same reflections for the fusion zones, but there is a discontinuity in the weld.

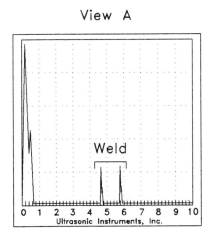
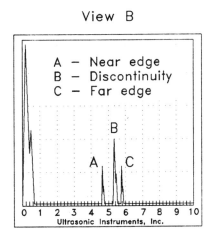

Suppose the display for this test does *not* show both fusion zones. Given the following problems, which do you think exists?

The sound beam does not penetrate the weld . . . . **Page 3-46**
Excessive porosity in the weld metal absorbs the
sound beam . . . . **Page 3-48**

That is right. If no indications are present it may be that the sound beam has not penetrated the weld, as in this example. Failure of penetration is not an uncommon occurrence. When it happens, you simply change the frequency and try again or you change the position or angle of the transducer.

In order to scan the welded seam over its entire cross section at one particular spot, you move the angle beam transducer forward and backward alternately approaching and moving away from the weld at a distance of one-half to one "skip distances" from the center of the weld seam. Moving the transducer forward and backward in this manner causes the entire weld to be scanned as illustrated below.

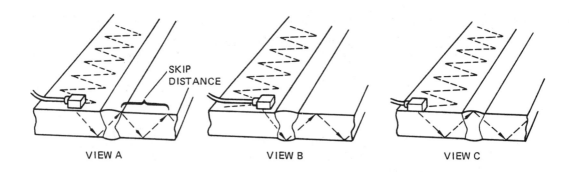

A reflection will be received from a discontinuity in the weld, even when the center of the beam does not strike it. The maximum reflection, however, will be received when the discontinuity is struck by the center of the beam.

False . . . . **Page 3-49**
True . . . . **Page 3-51**

The path of a shear wave from an angle beam transducer showing the "nodes" of the beam is illustrated below.

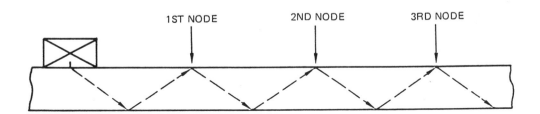

1ST NODE   2ND NODE   3RD NODE

The location of the nodes can be determined by finger damping or by rubbing with a couplant-filled brush away from or toward the transducer along the sound path. This action will interfere with reflections of sound when the hand or brush is at the nodes and the indications on the CRT will be dampened at the point of interference. In this way, the point where the sound strikes the surface is readily identified.

Skip distance can also be determined mathematically from:

Skip distance = 2 (thickness) x tan (refracted angle).

Skip distance, or the distance as measured on the surface between two nodes, can be determined by measuring the distance between two adjacent points that show reduced indications on the CRT. When the finger touches a point on the surface between two nodes, there will be no dampening of the sound wave.

Skip distance is a function of which of the following factors?

Frequency . . . . **Page 3-50**
Wedge angle . . . . **Page 3-52**

Your selection is not correct. Excessive porosity in the weld metal would not be the cause since there could be a reflection from the nearest fusion zone and reflections from the weld where the porosity occurs.

In this example, if you fail to receive indications that show both fusion zones, the sound beam has not penetrated through the weld. The sound beam either does not have the power required (in which case a lower frequency will help) or the beam is approaching the weld at such an angle that all of the beam is being reflected or scattered (in which case moving the transducer to another location may help).

Turn back to page 3-46.

Your selection is not correct. A sound beam is strongest in the center and grows progressively weaker as distance from the center increases. The reflection from a discontinuity will be strongest when the discontinuity is struck by the center of the beam, even though a small reflection *will* occur when it is struck by the weaker portion of the beam.

Turn ahead to page 3-51.

If you have turned to this page, it indicates you think skip distance is a function of the frequency of the sound wave being transmitted into the test specimen.

Consider now what determines the angle of sound in a material. Isn't the angle due to the angle of incidence of the sound beam on the test surface and the ratio of the velocity of sound in the wedge to that in the test specimen? It is. Since frequency isn't a factor to be considered in figuring the angle of refraction from Snell's Law, it is apparent that frequency is not the correct answer. The angle of incidence, as determined by the angle of the Lucite wedge, is the factor that determines skip distance.

Turn ahead to page 3-52.

Correct. A sound beam is strongest in the center. Maximum reflection from a discontinuity is received when it is struck by the center of the sound beam.

To use the proper scanning technique for welds, it is necessary to understand "skip distance" and the means for finding it.

But, hold up! Before turning back to page 3-47, take that coffee break, stretch your legs and relax. You're doing just fine!

That's right. Skip distance is determined by the refracted angle of the sound beam that propagates in the test specimen. This is determined by the incident angle of the Lucite (plexiglass) wedge.

Once the skip distance is known, the area over which the transducer is to be moved in scanning the weld can be determined by drawing or marking two reference points or lines parallel to the weld seam; one at one-half the skip distance and one at one skip distance from the center of the weld seam. With the aid of the center line on the probe, you can then move the transducer in a zigzag path from the weld toe to the reference mark at a full skip distance. The one-half skip distance mark can be used for one-half node examinations to completely scan the weld. Contact between the transducer and test surface must remain uniform throughout the scanning path, as spurious indications or loss of indications will result. And remember, we must watch the CRT and *not* the scanning motion as we move the probe.

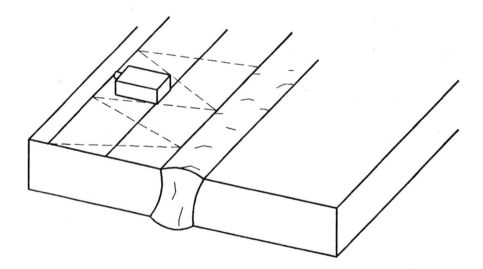

Turn to the next page.

Serious discontinuities in the weld seam, such as cracks and slag, usually extend longitudinally along the seam and give particularly clear indications when the sound beam strikes the joint at right angles.

Assuming the same wedge is used and the same material properties are maintained, will skip distance increase or decrease as thickness of the test specimen is increased?

Decrease . . . . **Page 3-54**
Increase . . . . **Page 3-56**

"Skip distance" will *not* decrease as the thickness of the test specimen is increased. The angle of refraction in the specimen will remain the same and the angles of reflection at the nodes will remain the same; however, as the thickness increases, the sound must travel further between nodes to the surface. As illustrated below, the correct answer is that the skip distance will *increase* as thickness of the test specimen is increased.

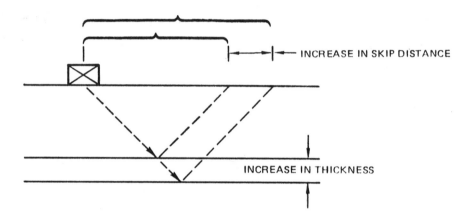

Turn ahead to page 3-56.

The statement is "false." As the thickness of the material is increased, the beam angle should be *decreased*. If not, the skip distance will increase and this creates problems in the sensitivity of the testing system. Remember, as the skip distance becomes greater, sensitivity decreases; therefore, in selecting an optimum beam angle in relation to material thickness, skip distance and attenuation must be taken into consideration.

Turn ahead to page 3-57.

Correct. Skip distance will *increase* as the thickness of the test specimen is increased. The angle of refraction in the test specimen will remain the same, but as the thickness is increased, the distance between nodes will increase.

Generally the refracted angle of the sound beam selected should be as large as practical when testing welds. Many testing codes dictate what angles can be used for weld testing, usually 45°, 60°, and 70°. The test procedure will also provide direction for the test at hand. At smaller beam angles, small spurious indications may be returned from the weld root or weld cap (crown) and these can be difficult to distinguish from real discontinuities. Smaller angles, however, must be used on thick plates to reduce the skip distance, as too great a skip distance will cause a reduction in the sensitivity of the test system.

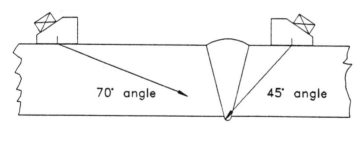
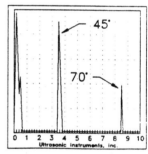

Judgment must be used in selecting a large angle of incidence for the generation of shear waves. What will happen if the angle selected is so large that the angle of refraction is 90°?

Skip distance will be too great .... **Page 3-58**
Surface waves will be produced .... **Page 3-60**

Good. You determined that the statement was false and you're correct. As material thickness increases, beam angle should be *decreased*. Otherwise skip distance and attenuation will increase, which will result in reduced test system sensitivity.

Let's see how the physical location of a discontinuity in a weld can be determined in angle beam testing. We know that the distance in the display represents the angle beam sound-path distance in the test specimen *plus* the distance the sound beam traveled through the transducer wedge.

The typical test procedure contains methods of calibrating that allow the operator to make these compensations easily. Calibrations are performed based on actual reflected signals with disregard to the placement of the initial pulse. In doing so, the "0" screen division truly represents the sound entry point on the test object.

Turn ahead to page 3-59.

Your selection is not the best. If the angle of refraction is 90°, surface waves are produced which are of little value in evaluating the internal (volumetric) condition of welds.

Surface waves are not able to penetrate very far below the surface of the material.

Turn ahead to page 3-60.

The distance "a" between the transducer and the discontinuity can be calculated according to the equation a = W (sin α) where α is the refracted angle and W is the length of the true beam path or sound path as illustrated below.

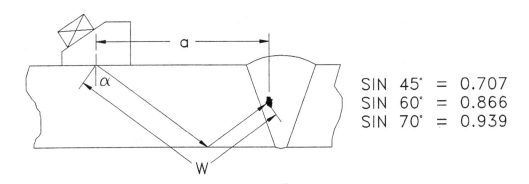

SIN 45° = 0.707
SIN 60° = 0.866
SIN 70° = 0.939

The equation tells us that to find a value for "a" we multiply the value for "W" by the sine of the beam angle.

In a practical test situation, assume you are testing a weld in a steel specimen at a beam angle of 60°. The sound-path distance "W," as measured on the CRT screen, is 7.9 inches (20.1 cm). What is the distance "a" from the centerline of the wedge angle to the discontinuity?

7 inches (17.8 cm) . . . . **Page 3-61**
7.9 inches (20.1 cm) . . . . **Page 3-64**

Excellent—if the angle of incidence becomes so great that the angle of refraction in the test specimen is 90°, shear waves will no longer be produced. Surface waves will result, and it is not possible to thoroughly test the volume of a weld with surface waves.

The following table provides a comparison of the most favorable beam angles for testing welds in materials of varying thickness, first with the weld caps flush with the material surface, and then with the weld caps not removed.

WELD CAPS FLUSH ON BOTH SIDES		
PLATE THICKNESS (INCHES)	BEAM ANGLE (DEGREES)	SKIP DISTANCE (INCHES)
0.2 - 0.6	80	2.2 - 6.6
0.6 - 1.2	70	3.2 - 6.6
1.2 - 2.4	60	4.2 - 8.4
OVER 2.4	45	4.8 AND UP
WELD CAPS NOT REMOVED		
0.2 - 0.8	80	2.2 - 8.8
0.8 - 1.6	70	4.4 - 8.8
OVER 1.6	60	5.6 AND UP

Is the following statement true or false? As plate thickness is increased, beam angle should be increased.

True .... **Page 3-55**
False .... **Page 3-57**

Excellent. The correct answer is 6.8 inches (17.3 cm) rounded to 7 inches (17.8 cm). You may find "W" by multiplying the total sound-path distance (7.9 inches or 20.1 cm) by the sine of 60° given as 0.866. The resultant distance "a" is the distance from the center line (or "exit point") of the wedge angle to a point directly above the discontinuity.

Turn to the next page.

Assume you are testing a weld in a steel specimen at an angle of 80°. One-half the skip distance has been determined to be 2 inches (50.8 mm). With the transducer at this position, a discontinuity indication appears on the CRT at the 4th major screen division. This will indicate that the discontinuity is at the root of the weld since at one-half the skip distance the sound beam strikes the root of the weld seam. (NOTE: At angles of 80°, the distance from the transducer to the discontinuity can, for all practical purposes, approximate the true sound path.)

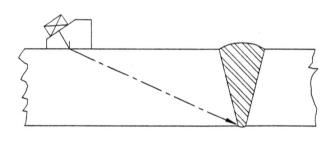 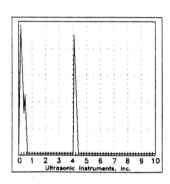

Now assume that while scanning the same weld, a discontinuity indication appears at the 3rd major screen division.

From the above assumption, where would you say the discontinuity is located?

Center of weld seam . . . . **Page 3-65**
Between the transducer and weld seam . . . . **Page 3-67**

No. The discontinuity *is in the weld*. By turning to this page you have indicated that you forgot to consider what the full skip distance mark is all about. Remember too that at an angle of 80° the angular path of the sound beam is considered to be essentially the same as the distance measured parallel to the surface. Since the transducer is at the whole skip distance, the discontinuity must be located in the center line of the weld.

Turn ahead to page 3-69.

We suspect that you took a quick guess on this one. Guessing is easier than working it out. If you did guess, then you're in trouble, since there is no room for guessing in nondestructive testing. You have to know!

We gave you the equation a = W (sin α) which tells you that you can find the value for "a" by multiplying the value for "W" by the sine of the refracted beam angle.

The true value for "W" is the same as the sound-path distance that is read on the CRT. Since the distance read on the CRT was 7.9 inches (20.1 cm), the value for "W" is 7.9 inches (20.1 cm).

Since the beam angle is 60°, then from the table the sine of 60° is 0.866.

Now, 7.9 inches (20.1 cm) times 0.866 is equal to 6.8 inches (17.3 cm) or practically *7 inches (17.8 cm)*.

Turn back to page 3-61.

You did not select the correct answer. This discontinuity is *not* located at the center of the weld seam.

You may have forgotten that the 4th major screen division is the root and, in this case, the center of the weld.

The illustration below explains the situation.

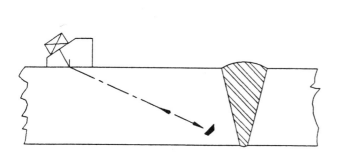

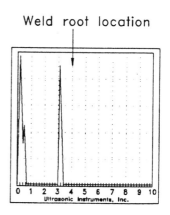

Weld root location

If the weld root appears at the location pointed out, the indication to the left of this position *must* occur *before* the weld root.

This discontinuity is, in fact, between the transducer and the weld. Can you now see why?

Turn ahead to page 3-67.

Not quite.   The "first leg" was defined as the *actual sound path* associated with the 1/2 skip distance.   Therefore, the first leg is that portion of the propagating sound beam beneath and extending beyond the search unit.

Note the first leg indicated on the illustration again and review your response.

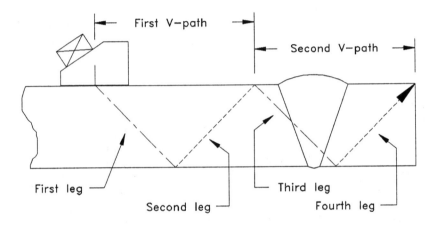

Turn ahead to page 3-70.

Good. If the weld root appears at the 4th major screen division, any indication to the left of this position *must* occur *before* the weld root.

Next, a discontinuity indication on the CRT appears at the 8th major screen division. This will indicate that the discontinuity is in the plate beyond the weld as illustrated.

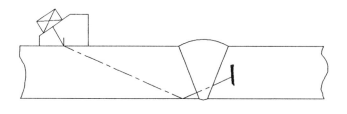 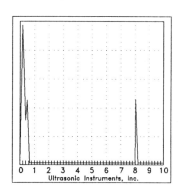

During scanning, the center line of the wedge on the transducer is at the whole skip distance mark when a discontinuity indication appears. The discontinuity is:

beyond the weld . . . . **Page 3-63**
in the weld . . . . **Page 3-69**

Your answer is incorrect. Note the location of the discontinuity. It is at the boundary between the specimen and the weld metal. In this case the discontinuity is caused by a *lack of fusion* between the specimen and the weld which will cause the weld to be weakened. *Lack of penetration* is caused by molten weld material not flowing throughout the area to be filled at the weld root.

Turn ahead to page 3-78.

An excellent choice! The discontinuity is in the weld. At 80° the angular path of the sound beam is considered to be the same as the distance measured parallel to the surface.

We should point out a couple of other terms before we move on in our contact angle beam discussion. The "first leg" is the descriptor used to define the *actual sound path* associated with the one-half skip distance. Odd numbers are sequentially assigned to multiples of this sound-path trajectory. The "second leg" describes the *actual sound path* of the rest of the first skip distance on the return to the examination surface. The total *sound-path distance traveled* in a skip distance is the "V-path." Refer to the illustration below for a closer look at these new terms.

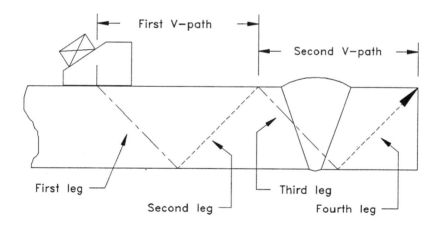

In the illustration above, which leg is traveling through the weld?

First leg **3-66**
Third leg **3-70**

Bravo! We just defined the term and you've got it already.

It should now be more evident than ever that angle beam testing carries a bit of math, a pinch of new terms, and a spoonful of logic to reason out the most probable sound path within the material.

Assume now that you have available an International Institute of Welding (IIW) ultrasonic reference block for use in calibrating the instrument for testing welds in steel. You will recall that the IIW block was described in detail in Volume II.

Turn to the next page and let's get calibrated!

In general, instrument calibration for angle beam testing of welds in steel using the IIW block (Type I) is accomplished as follows:

●   After the instrument completes its self-test, connect the probe to the instrument. Adjust the delay such that the initial pulse is located near the "0" screen division. Adjust the range for approximately a 10.0 inch (25.4 cm) FSW. Increase the gain until a slight baseline noise is present.

●   Next we must determine the "exit point" of sound from the plexiglass wedge. Position the probe as illustrated below and maximize the indication from the 4-inch (10.2 cm) radius by sliding the probe back and forth. Note the curve on the CRT that the signal follows or traces as you move the probe. The CRT position of the indication is unimportant at this point. A gain adjustment may be necessary to see the top of the indication. Mark the wedge just above the 4-inch (10.2 cm) radius indication on the IIW block.

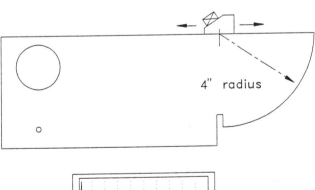

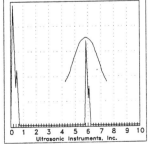

Turn to the next page.

- Position the search unit near the refracted angle indications on the IIW block that correspond to the angle of the wedge. The illustration indicates the general idea. Maximize the response from the plexiglass insert in the IIW block and read the refracted angle immediately below to the exit point mark defined in step 2. Again, its precise CRT position is unimportant.

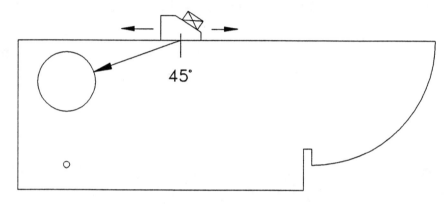

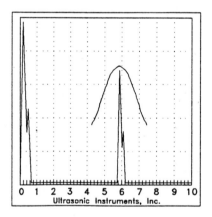

Turn to the next page.

● Place the probe back to the position in which the 4-inch (10.2 cm) radius was maximized (step 2). Peak the indication and position it to the 4th screen division with the delay. Adjust the range so that a second indication appears at the 9th screen division. These adjustments affect one another, so repeat the process until the CRT appears as illustrated, a 10 inch (25.4 cm) FSW. Again, gain adjustments may be required.

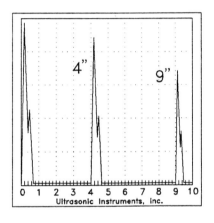

10" FSW

● Finally, position the probe to maximize the 0.060-inch (1.5 mm) side-drilled hole and adjust the peak of this indication to 80% FSH with the gain control. This establishes the test sensitivity.

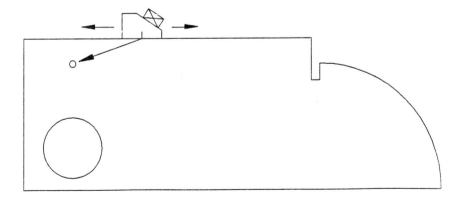

Turn to the next page.

This brings us now to the use of the direct reading ultrasonic calculator for weld testing when the plate thickness of the test specimen and angle of the transducer are known. Cards similar to that shown below are available commercially, or can be easily made with transparent paper and graph paper and are quite handy to use.

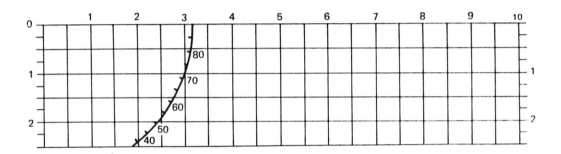

The horizontal scale across the top of the card represents the number of inches between the transducer and the weld. The vertical scale represents specimen thickness and the numbers adjacent to the arc show the refracted angle of the sound beam. A transparent, plastic slide fits over the card and is used to identify the weld and show its location in the specimen. A typical example using this form of calculator follows.

Turn to the next page.

Assume now that we are testing a double-V groove weld in a 2 inch (50.8 mm) steel plate. The transducer we're using has a 60° refracted angle in steel.

- First, we draw a line representing the sound path from the upper left corner of the card (representing point of entry in the specimen) through the 60° mark on the arc as shown below. The line should extend to the 2 inch (50.8 mm) line (point A) representing plate thickness. We now have the sound beam angle recorded on the card. The angled line also represents one-half the skip distance as measured on the surface—approximately 3-7/16 inches (87.3 mm).

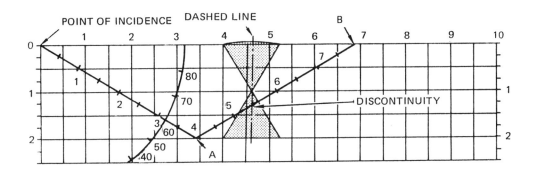

- For full skip distance, we double the 3-7/16 inches (87.3 mm) and mark that point at approximately 6-7/8 inches or 17.5 cm (point B). We then draw a line between point A and point B and mark off the two lines in inches as shown above. The scale should be the same as the horizontal and vertical lines on the card.
- We then sketch the 30° weld on the plastic slide, with the dashed line representing the exact center of the weld, and place the card in the slide.

Turn to the next page.

● Now let's assume that the instrument CRT shows a discontinuity at a sound path of 5-5/8 inches (14.3 cm) when the center line of the transducer (point of incidence) is 4-5/8 inches (11.7 cm) from the weld center line. First we locate the plastic slide weld center line over the 4-5/8 inch (11.7 cm) mark on the card. Then the discontinuity location is read directly by reading along the sound path to a point 5-5/8 inches (14.3 cm) from the point of sound entry. We find the discontinuity is 1-1/4 inches (31.8 mm) from the surface and 1/8 inch (3.2 mm) from the center of the weld on the far side of the weld.

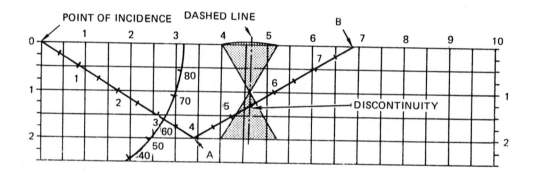

Which of the following discontinuities is apparent in the above example?

Lack of penetration . . . . Page 3-68
Lack of fusion . . . . Page 3-78

Incorrect. In this example the discontinuity is located at the lower part of the single-V groove weld where the two sections of the specimen are joined. The discontinuity is caused by *lack of penetration* of the molten weld material into this space and not by lack of fusion between the weld material and specimen.

Turn ahead to page 3-80.

That's right. The indicated discontinuity is caused by a lack of fusion between the edge of the specimen and the weld.

Assume now that we're testing a single-V groove weld in a 1-inch-thick (25.4 mm) steel specimen. The transducer wedge angle is 70°.

●   The sound path is drawn on the card from the upper left corner toward the 70° mark on the arc and down to the horizontal line at 1 inch (point A) as shown below. For the full skip distance we double the length of this line and place a mark at approximately 5-1/2 inches or 13.9 cm (point B). The second half of the sound path is then drawn in.

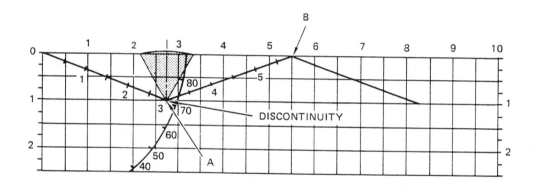

●   We add the inch (or mm) scale to the sound path as we did in the previous example, sketch the weld on the transparent, plastic slide, and place the prepared card in the slide.

Turn to the next page.

Refer to the adjacent page and continue:

● Let's now assume a discontinuity indication at 3 inches (76.2 mm) on the CRT screen when the transducer point of incidence is 2-3/4 inches (69.9 mm) from the weld center line. We adjust the weld center line on the plastic slide over the 2-3/4 mark on the card and read the location of the discontinuity directly by reading along the sound path to a point 3 inches (76.2 mm) from the point of incidence. The discontinuity occurs 1 inch (25.4 mm) below the surface and in the center of the weld.

Which of the following discontinuities is apparent in the above examples?

Lack of fusion .... **Page 3-77**
Lack of penetration .... **Page 3-80**

Very good. The indicated discontinuity is caused by *lack of penetration* of the molten material at the root of the weld.

The experienced ultrasonic operator can determine the type of discontinuity from the location, shape, and response of an indication in the display. Typical indications from the common discontinuities are as follows:

- Cracks and bonding discontinuities in the direction of the weld seam will produce a sharply-defined indication when the beam strikes at right angles.
- Porosity that is spherical in shape will produce a sharp echo even when the beam strikes at an angle to the weld seam.
- Slag streaks produce a stepped indication that is maximum at right angles to the weld seam. This discontinuity differs but little from cracks with flat surfaces.

Turn ahead to page 3-84.

A typical application of the technique is in sizing or assessing a crack's height as measured from the inside of the component toward the outside or vice versa. From the illustration, we can see that a signal will be reflected at the base of the crack (B). Likewise, a tip diffracted signal will be generated at the tip (T) as long as the crack height does not exceed the beam spread. For deeper cracks, we simply move the search unit until we maximize the tip signal, though characterizing the tip signal in this fashion can be a challenge, even for the most experienced technicians.

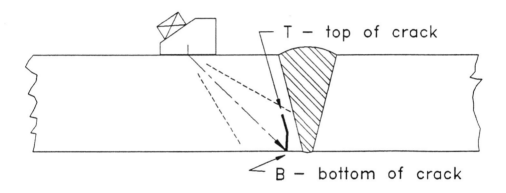

Would you think it possible to determine the through-wall dimension of a crack on the _examination side_ of a plate using a two transducer technique?

Sure **3-87**

No way **3-88**

Good. The transducer should be placed at the minimum and maximum points in distance from the center line of the reference hole—the same distance that will be used later in scanning the test specimen.

Let's consider one final technique. "Tip diffraction" is a technique useful for establishing the extremities of cracks that propagate through the thickness of plates, pipes, and vessels. The concept is to take advantage of the signal generated from the tip of the flaw as it *diffracts or bends* the sound beam passing over or under it. Notice in the illustration below, that the bending of the incident beam results in a wave that propagates from the top or tip of the notch. This signal locates the end point of the crack and defines its through-wall dimension. We will stick with contact pulse echo approaches of the technique to simplify things a bit except for one example.

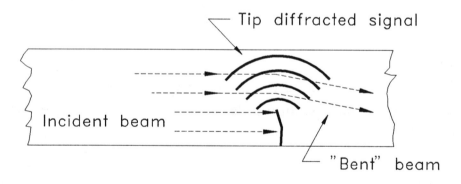

Turn back to page 3-81.

Your answer is not the most practical solution to the problem since it may require the selection of several different angles before one can be found that will give the proper discontinuity indication. It will be much better to test from the other side of the weld seam to see if unfavorable multiple reflections can be avoided.

In the event that testing from the other side of the seam also results in multiple reflections, it may then be necessary to experiment and use different angles in an attempt to obtain a definable discontinuity indication.

Turn ahead to page 3-86.

- A large inclusion can produce multiple reflections with interference by reflections from the surface of the plate.

These CRT responses are illustrated below along with a cross section of a large inclusion.

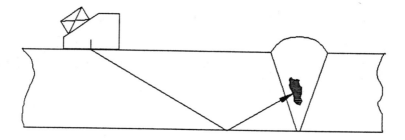

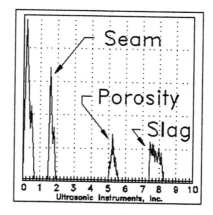

Ultrasonic Instruments, Inc.

If a multiple reflection is received from a discontinuity such as the large inclusion in the illustration above, what would be the best way to isolate its location?

Test with different beam angle .... **Page 3-83**
Test from other side of weld seam .... **Page 3-86**

Stop and think a bit. The function of a reference standard is to provide indication data to which indications of discontinuities may be compared. Therefore, isn't it reasonable to test the reference standard in the same way that we intend to test the weld? You bet it is.

The magnitude of the reflections obtained from the hole in the reference standard should be determined from the minimum and maximum points to be included in the scanning path when actually testing the weld. This will normally be with the probe at the toe of the weld and at the full skip distance. Skip distance, of course, is a function of the angle of the sound beam incidence on the test surface and the thickness of the test specimen.

To obtain the magnitude of reflection only from the mid-point of the area of scan would not provide adequate reference information since this is only one of the very large number of possible test locations on the test item.

Turn back to page 3-82.

Excellent. The most practical solution to the problem is to test from the other side of the weld seam first. If this procedure also results in multiple reflections, then additional beam angles may be applied.

Ideally, the reference standard to use for comparison in weld inspection is a welded sample of the same type and size as that being tested. The reference standard should contain known discontinuities of the same size and type as those suspected in the test specimen. However, this type of comparative standard is difficult to obtain in practical test situations. As an alternative, it is common practice to place a side-drilled hole in the test specimen or in a separate piece of similar material of the same general size and compare reflections from this hole with reflections received from discontinuities in the test specimen.

The hole size commonly used is 1/16 inch (1.6 mm) in diameter by 1/2 to 2 inches (12.7 to 50.8 mm) deep. The actual size of the hole, or in some cases, notch, to be used as a reference standard will be prescribed by the test procedure.

If you are determining the magnitude of the reflection that will be received from the hole in the reference standard, at what distance should the transducer be placed from the hole?

Minimum and maximum for weld scanning . . . . **Page 3-82**
Mid-point of area of scan . . . . **Page 3-85**

Absolutely! That is how the technique was first applied. (Turn to page 3-88 for an illustration.)

Although the technique applies well to shear waves, it also applies to longitudinal waves. In longitudinal wave applications, the operator can locate the crack tip on the opposite side of the weld itself. Note the following figure.

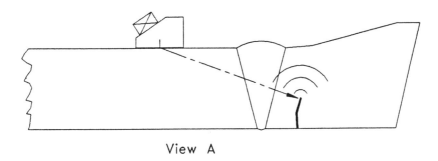

View A

"High angle" longitudinal waves, which propagate at refracted angles from about 60° to 85°, can detect the tip signals generated by cracks that extend almost through-wall. But, don't forget that this means shear waves will also be propagating into the test article creating potential signal interpretation headaches for the operator. We referred to this as "bi-modal" earlier in the chapter.

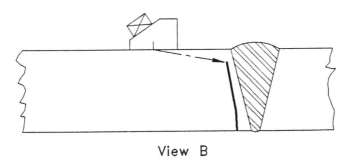

View B

Turn ahead to page 3-89.

Oh, but there is a way! The technique was first developed for this very purpose. Take a look at the figure below. Because the tip signal propagates in a radial fashion, it will reach the receiving transducer. Using a little of that math and logic you possess, you can determine the through-wall extent of the signal based on "time-of-flight" to the receiving probe.

Path of tip diffracted signal

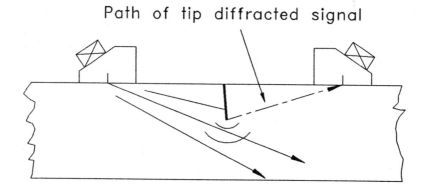

Turn back to page 3-87.

Applications in which tip diffraction is useful include:

• Sizing of under clad cracking in pressure vessels and piping.
• Determination of through-wall dimension of cracks in pipe that has been overlayed with multilayers of weld material.
• Determination of the size or diameter of porosity in welds, composites, and ceramics.

Calibration for tip diffraction requires a reference block that contains notches ranging from 10% to 90% through-wall in 10% increments. The calibration is done in terms of depth (from the examination surface to the top of the discontinuity) as opposed to the sound-path distance we discussed earlier when calibrating with the IIW block. Essentially, as the notch height *increases*, the time-of-flight for the tip signal *decreases*. Therefore the tip signal arrives earlier in time or closer to the initial pulse.

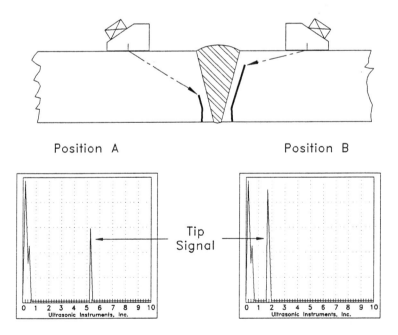

Turn to the next page.

Put on your thinking cap and review the illustration below and then answer the question that follows.

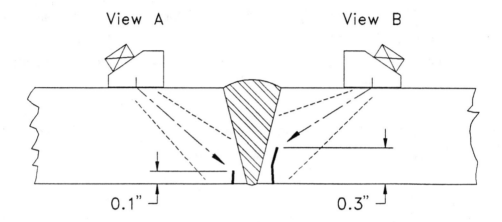

Given that you will receive both an inside corner trap signal AND a tip diffracted signal, which view above will result in the _greatest_ separation between the signals?

View A **3-91**
View B **3-92**

No. The corner trap signal will *always* appear at the same location. With a depth calibration, that location will equate to the thickness of the plate or test article. The only indication that will move will be the tip signal. It will move closer to the initial pulse as the crack height *increases.* Review the accompanying CRT's below .

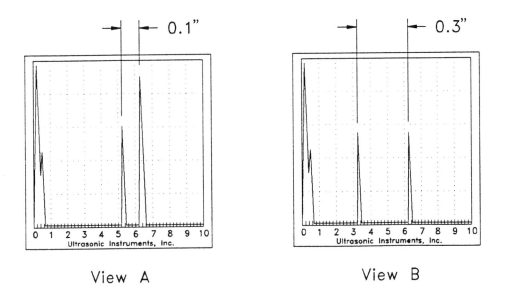

View A

View B

Turn to the next page.

Well done! You immediately realized that the corner trap signal will always appear at the same location and that is the screen position representing the thickness of the plate or test article. The only indication that will move will be the tip signal. It will move closer to the initial pulse as the crack height increases. The CRT presentations are shown below to illustrate the point.

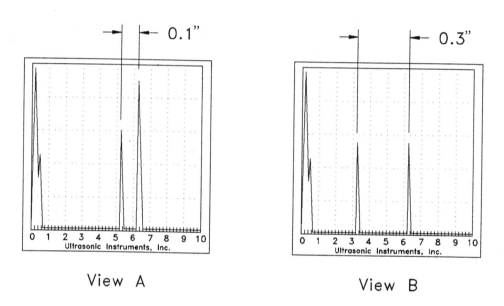

View A   View B

Wow! You've worked hard to get through this much information in a single chapter. Take a stretch break, reread any concepts you're confused about, and turn to the next page for a chapter review.

CHAPTER REVIEW

_____   1.   Given a choice of the following transducer frequencies for testing a casting, the most practical selection is the _____ MHz transducer.

A.   1.0
B.   2.0
C.   5.0
D.   25.0

_____   2.   Knowledge of probable orientation of discontinuities in test specimens is important to the ultrasonic operator. Discontinuities in forgings are likely to be oriented _____ to the direction of working.

A.   perpendicular
B.   crosswise
C.   parallel
D.   Any of the above.

_____   3.   In testing bar stock from the end, discontinuities can still exist in the bar and not cause reflections if they are oriented _____ to the length of the bar.

A.   perpendicular
B.   oblique
C.   crosswise
D.   parallel

_____ 4. In a diametrical inspection of bar stock, sound transmission can be improved using a transducer having a _____ that fits the radius of the bar.

   A. bent shoe
   B. frequency flat
   C. velocity
   D. curved shoe

_____ 5. Initial examination of large plate with a straight beam transducer should be conducted by performing a _____ scan.

   A. gross
   B. detailed

_____ 6. Discontinuities in rolled plate are likely to be oriented _____ the surface.

   A. perpendicular to
   B. crosswise with
   C. parallel to
   D. mirrored to

_____ 7. When testing plate materials, the discontinuities are sometimes compared with reflections received from a _____ of given dimensions called out in the test procedure.

    A. slag inclusion
    B. reference notch
    C. undercut
    D. stringer

_____ 8. A plate should be scanned from at least _____ faces to reduce the effect of "skip distance" that overlooks some discontinuities.

    A. two
    B. three
    C. four
    D. eight

_____ 9. The most flexible transducer to select for generation of plate waves in a thin plate is one that has a(n) _____ angle.

    A. fixed
    B. rotated
    C. variable
    D. inverted

10. A (an) _____ beam transducer is extremely valuable in pinpointing discontinuities in rolled sheet and plate and for making gross checks.

   A. straight
   B. angle
   C. variable-fixed
   D. surface wave

11. A (an) _____ transducer should be selected to conduct an ultrasonic test on a welded section of 6-inch (15.2 cm) pipe.

   A. straight beam
   B. rotated beam
   C. variable beam
   D. angle beam

12. For generating surface waves, the ultrasonic operator needs an angle beam transducer with a wedge angle that lies beyond the:

   A. first critical.
   B. near zone.
   C. far field.
   D. second critical angle.

_____ 13. With a transducer in a fixed position during ultrasonic testing of a pipe, some discontinuities may be overlooked by the sound beam as it travels around the pipe's circumference due to skip distance. This can be overcome by _____ the pipe from end to end.

    A. varying
    B. scanning
    C. oscillating
    D. flattening

_____ 14. The actual sound-path distance for a full skip distance is known as the:

    A. V-path.
    B. first leg.
    C. third leg.
    D. wedge delay.

_____ 15. During pipe testing, the distance from the transducer to a discontinuity can be measured on the CRT by utilizing the _____ screen divisions.

    A. horizontal
    B. vertical
    C. diagonal
    D. elongated

16. Standards are prepared for pipe and tubing by machining reference _____ on the inside and outside diameters of a sample of either the test specimen or other specimen of the same ultrasonic qualities.

A. circles
B. notches
C. biscuits
D. widgets

17. The _____ in a weld between base metal and weld material may cause reflections on the CRT even though there are no discontinuities present.

A. slag
B. lack of penetration
C. fusion zone
D. porosity

18. The maximum reflection from a discontinuity is received when the discontinuity is struck by the _____ of the sound beam.

A. top
B. center
C. left edge
D. back

_____   19.   Skip distance in a test specimen will change as the angle of _____ is changed.

              A.   reflection
              B.   oscillation
              C.   refraction
              D.   proportion

_____   20.   It is desirable to use large angles of incidence for the generation of shear waves. However, judgment must be used, since surface waves may be produced when the angle of refraction of shear waves in the test specimen exceeds:

              A.   45°.
              B.   60°.
              C.   70°.
              D.   90°.

_____   21.   A relationship exists between the thickness of a test specimen and the most desirable sound beam angle in the specimen. As the thickness of the test specimen is increased, the sound beam angle should be:

              A.   increased.
              B.   left unchanged.
              C.   decreased.

_____ 22. Assume you are testing a weld at an angle of 60°. A discontinuity appears at the 7th major screen division. This distance is _____ than the distance between the wedge center line and a point on the surface directly above the discontinuity.

A. less
B. greater
C. the same as

_____ 23. During weld scanning at 60°, a discontinuity indication appears when the transducer is 3 inches (76.2 mm) from the center of the weld seam which appears at the 4th screen division. The weld root indication appears at the 5th major screen division. Is the discontinuity located in the weld seam or in the plate?

A. Neither. It is in the wedge.
B. Weld
C. Plate

_____ 24. Assume you have angle beam transducers available that will produce angles of 60°, 70° and 80° in a test specimen. One of these, the _____ transducer, will produce a beam that travels very nearly the same distance in the material as distance measured on the surface.

A. 80°
B. 70°
C. 60°
D. 45°

_____ 25. International Institute of Welding (IIW) steel reference blocks are used for calibrating ultrasonic instruments for testing welds in:

    A. steel.
    B. aluminum.
    C. composites.
    D. ceramics.

_____ 26. A hole drilled in a test specimen is to be used as a reference standard for comparison with discontinuity indications from a weld. In establishing reference indications from the test hole, the transducer should be moved within the limits that will be used in _____ the weld.

    A. plotting
    B. scanning
    C. extrapolating
    D. machining

_____ 27. The term "tip diffraction" has been applied to mean the signal generated by the _____ of the sound beam caused by the extremity of a discontinuity in its path.

    A. focusing
    B. warping
    C. bending
    D. spreading

_____   28.   Tip diffraction applies to two types of wave modes. However, only the _____ waves should be used to penetrate the weld and size cracks on the opposite side.

          A.   surface
          B.   plate
          C.   shear
          D.   longitudinal

_____   29.   In the illustration below, which CRT displays the crack tip signal with the greatest through-wall dimension?

          A.   View A
          B.   View B

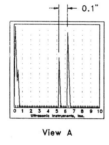 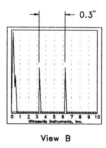

          View A   View B

Turn to the next page for answers to these review questions.

ANSWERS TO REVIEW QUESTIONS
FOR CHAPTER 3

Question & Answer		Reference Page(s)
1.	A	3-1, 3-5
2.	D	3-2, 3-4
3.	D	3-8
4.	D	3-8
5.	A	3-12, 3-16
6.	C	3-15
7.	B	3-22
8.	A	3-23
9.	C	3-30
10.	A	3-13, 3-16
11.	D	3-29, 3-35
12.	D	3-26
13.	B	3-33, 3-35
14.	A	3-69
15.	B	3-7, 3-62
16.	B	3-40
17.	C	3-45
18.	B	3-51
19.	C	3-47
20.	D	3-60

Question & Answer		Reference Page(s)
21.	C	3-56
22.	B	3-59
23.	C	3-62
24.	A	3-62
25.	A	3-70
26.	B	3-82
27.	C	3-82
28.	D	3-87
29.	B	3-92

Turn to the next page and begin Chapter 4.

CHAPTER 4

PULSE ECHO/THROUGH-TRANSMISSION TESTING USING THE IMMERSION TECHNIQUE

In Chapters 2 and 3 you learned about the application of contact testing and the various techniques that are used to properly evaluate discontinuity indications. Many of these applications and techniques are also used in immersion testing. Therefore, this chapter on immersion testing will cover only the equipment and techniques peculiar to immersion testing and the indications that may be expected when conducting tests. Little additional discussion will be given when the principles of the techniques are similar or identical to those discussed in contact testing.

You recall that in immersion testing the transducer is separated from the test surface of the test specimen by a liquid, usually water with a wetting agent and corrosion inhibitor added. In addition, under normal testing applications, both the test specimen and transducer are immersed in a tank and the ultrasound must pass through a short distance of liquid before reaching the surface of the test specimen.

Turn to the next page.

The equipment required in immersion testing depends upon the particular testing problem or application. A typical installation will include the following items.

- An ultrasonic test system, usually including a computer and a color printer
- A test tank to hold the coupling medium (water) and the test specimen
- A scanner tube for holding the transducer
- A manipulator for positioning the transducer
- A carriage to support the manipulator and permit movement of the transducer back and forth and across the test tank in any direction
- A turntable to permit rotation of symmetrically-shaped specimens for automatic scanning

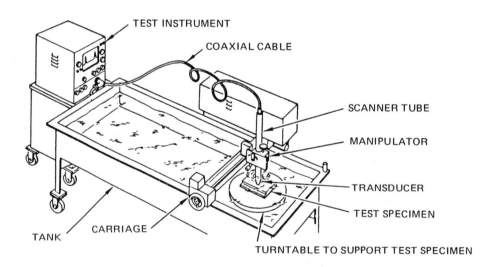

Water used in test tanks as a couplant usually requires the addition of a wetting agent. The wetting agent serves the purpose of:

elimination of air bubbles . . . . **Page 4-4**
aerating the water . . . . **Page 4-6**

Sorry, the manipulator is used to tilt the transducer to change the angle of incidence of the sound beam.

In order to determine the extent of the discontinuity, the transducer has to be moved back and forth along the surface of the test article. This is the function of the manual positioner.

Turn ahead to page 4-7.

Good. The "wetting agent" is added to the water in the test tank to reduce the surface tension and minimize air bubbles. We can expect the maximum transfer of ultrasonic energy into the test specimen when there are fewest obstructions to the passage of the sound beam—air bubbles are a definite obstruction.

Before considering the test frequencies that can be used in immersion testing, let's briefly review some of the basic equipment used in immersion testing.

The carriage assembly mounts on the immersion test tank and provides a means of moving the transducer in both longitudinal and transverse directions relative to the surface of the test specimen. The unit may be either manually or automatically operated. A manual unit is illustrated below.

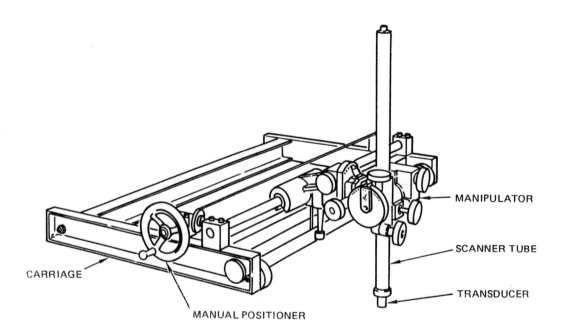

Turn to the next page.

Automatically-operated carriage units include a motor and drive mechanisms for moving and/or incrementing the transducer across the width and length of the tank to scan the entire surface. Speed of scanning is variable and is controlled by the operator.

Which of the following items should you adjust if you want to determine the extent of the area of a large discontinuity?

Manipulator . . . . **Page 4-3**
Manual positioner . . . . **Page 4-7**

No, no. If you were to "aerate" the water, its effectiveness as a couplant would be reduced, since ultrasound has just as much trouble getting through an air bubble in water as it has in getting through free air.

Your selection should have been "elimination of air bubbles." When there are no air bubbles in the water that surrounds a test specimen, the water "wets" the surface better and we have a better transfer of ultrasound from the water to the test specimen.

Turn back to page 4-4.

Fine. You are quite right. The *manual positioner* is used when you want to adjust the position of the transducer parallel to the test surface.

The "manipulator," you'll recall, is used to precisely raise, lower, or change the angle of the transducer with reference to the test surface of a specimen. The unit is so designed that, once set, the transducer position will be accurately maintained during scanning.

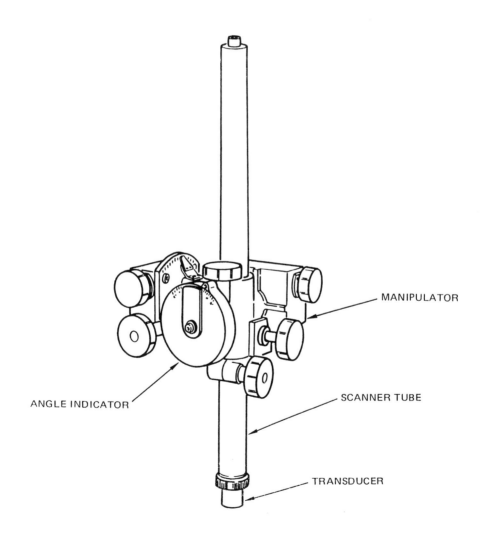

MANIPULATOR

ANGLE INDICATOR

SCANNER TUBE

TRANSDUCER

Turn to the next page.

In contact testing you learned that the angle imprinted on a Lucite wedge used in angle beam testing is conventionally the angle of refraction in a given test material, not the angle of incidence.

Which of the following angles do you think is shown by the angle indicator on the manipulator?

Angle of incidence at test surface . . . . **Page 4-10**
Angle of refraction in test specimen . . . . **Page 4-12**

That's right. The scanner tube is moved vertically to change the water distance between the transducer and test specimen by adjusting the manipulator.

Now let's consider the test frequencies that may be used in immersion testing.

Since the transducer does not come into contact with the test specimen in immersion testing, it is possible to use thinner crystals and thus test at the higher ultrasonic frequencies.

As in contact testing, the nature of the internal structure of the test specimen and the size of the discontinuity expected will be major factors in determining the frequency to be used. Where the test situation permits, it is possible to use frequencies as high as 15, 20, or 25 MHz. The frequency range of test instruments used in immersion testing is usually from 2.25 to 25 MHz.

Suppose the purpose of an ultrasonic test is to detect very small discontinuities. You have a choice of 10 MHz or 20 MHz as a test frequency.

Which should be selected for the best detectability of small discontinuities?

10 MHz . . . . **Page 4-11**
20 MHz . . . . **Page 4-14**

Correct. The angle shown by the angle indicator in the manipulator is the *angle of incidence* at the surface of the test specimen.

The scanner tube with the manipulator, shown on page 4-7, provides a rigid coaxial connection with a watertight mount on one end for the transducer and a standard coaxial connector on the other end. Scanner tubes are provided in varying lengths as indicated by test requirements.

Which element of the immersion testing system is raised or lowered to adjust the water distance between the transducer and the test specimen?

Scanner tube . . . . **Page 4-9**
Carriage . . . . **Page 4-13**

You picked the wrong answer. If you want to detect the smallest discontinuity, select the highest frequency available. The higher frequency will provide a sound beam of the shortest wavelength—the shorter the wavelength, the smaller the discontinuity that the beam can "see" or detect.

The sound beam can "see" a much smaller discontinuity at 20 MHz than at 10 MHz.

Turn ahead to page 4-14.

Incorrect. The angle shown on the angle indicator portion of the manipulator is the angle of the sound beam in the water medium or the *angle of incidence* at the test surface. It is then necessary to apply Snell's Law or use a calculating device to calculate the angle of refraction in the test specimen. If the angle indicator showed the angle of refraction in the test specimen, it would be necessary to change the scale on the indicator each time a specimen of a different material was tested.

Turn back to page 4-10.

No, the carriage is not raised and lowered to adjust the water distance. We raise and lower the *scanner tube* by adjusting the manipulator.

Remember, it is the manipulator that is adjusted to raise, lower, or change the angle of the scanner tube. It is the scanner tube that holds the transducer.

Turn back to page 4-9.

Very good. If you want to detect very small discontinuities and you have a choice between a test frequency of 10 MHz and 20 MHz, the 20 MHz frequency will give the best results when looking for small discontinuities.

Transducers used in immersion testing differ from those used in contact testing, mainly in the manner of construction. Since the transducer is immersed in water during testing, it follows that the transducer must be watertight. You have already learned that it is possible to make the transducer crystal much thinner for immersion testing since the transducer does not come into contact with the test specimen and therefore is not as susceptible to mechanical damage. The thinner crystal makes the higher test frequencies possible.

Turn to the next page.

For immersion testing applications where a sharper (or narrower) than normal sound beam is required, a *focused transducer* should be used. Focusing the sound beam will improve detectability of small discontinuities at any given frequency and will enable a search for discontinuities located at a given depth below the test surface. This type of transducer is especially useful in testing an area for satisfactory bonding between two materials.

The focusing effect, illustrated below, is attained by the structure of the acoustical lens on the face of the crystal. The lens focuses the sound energy into a small, well-defined pattern.

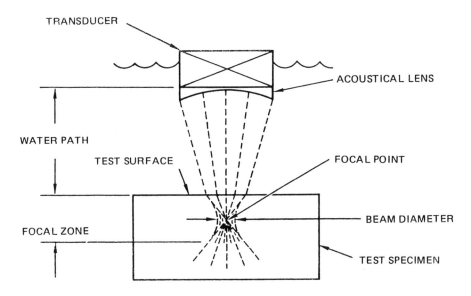

Turn to the next page.

Assume that you are testing by using a focused transducer with the results displayed on an A-scan device. Sweep delay is adjusted to "erase" the initial pulse. Further, assume that there are no discontinuities in the focal zone (sound path) of the transducer. **Which of the following indications will be displayed on the CRT?**

Front surface reflection only .... **Page 4-18**
Front surface and back surface reflection .... **Page 4-20**

As with any through-transmission setup, the transducers have to be properly aligned. A partial test setup showing the expected test instrument readout with proper and improper transducer alignment is shown below.

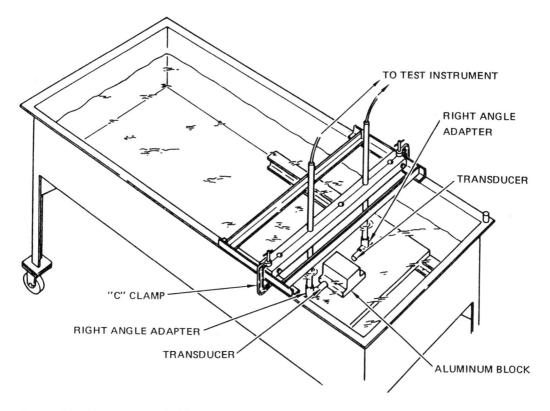

Turn ahead to page 4-19.

Very good. When using a focused transducer where no discontinuity exists within the focal zone of the transducer, no reflection will be returned for display on the CRT following the front surface indication.

Through-transmission techniques in immersion testing use the same "shadow" effects for detection of discontinuities as through-transmission techniques in contact testing. Maximum transmission of energy is obtained when there are no discontinuities in the test specimen—discontinuities cause reflection of the sound beam with a corresponding reduction of sound energy that is received by the receiving transducer. Accessory equipment for through-transmission testing is the same as for single-transducer techniques with the addition of a holding fixture for the second transducer. This can be either a second manipulator or, if one is not available, a holding fixture similar to this illustration.

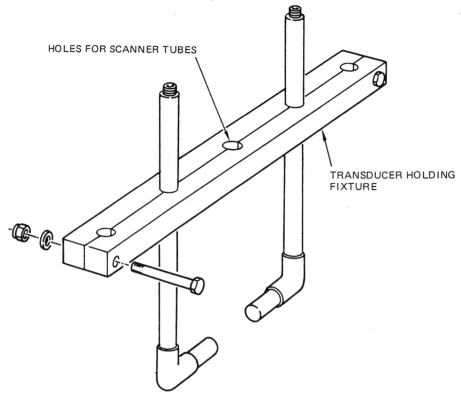

HOLES FOR SCANNER TUBES

TRANSDUCER HOLDING FIXTURE

Turn back to page 4-17.

Properly aligned   Improperly aligned

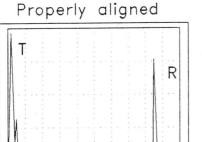
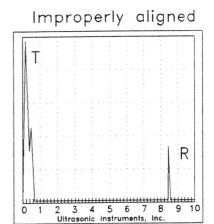

T — Transmitted pulse
R — Received pulse

What is the relationship between the size of a discontinuity and the amplitude of the received pulse on the CRT? Select one of the following.

Small discontinuity - small indication . . . . **Page 4-22**
Large discontinuity - small indication . . . . **Page 4-24**

Sorry. You made an incorrect selection. Under the stated hypothetical situation, the sound beam will diverge (scatter) beyond the focal zone of the transducer and there will be considerable scatter at the back surface. There will be very little, if any, energy returned from the back surface to cause an indication. A test under these conditions will result in only a *front surface indication*.

Turn back to page 4-18.

A variation of the "bubbler" is the high-temperature bubbler shown below that can be used for testing on surfaces that are too hot for standard contact testing. The flowing column of water insulates the transducer against heat and couples the sound beam to the test specimen.

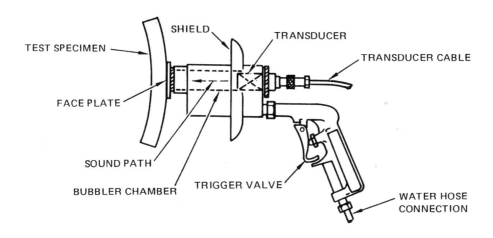

Which of the following can be considered an advantage in using a bubbler?

Both straight and angle beam techniques can be used . . Page 4-23
No immersion test tank is required . . . . Page 4-26

Your selection is not correct. If the discontinuity is small, more of the sound energy gets past and a larger amount will reach the receiving transducer. The indication of the received pulse on the CRT will be larger with a small discontinuity.

On the other hand, if the discontinuity is large, more of the sound beam will be reflected and less will pass through the specimen to the receiving transducer.

A good rule to remember in through-transmission testing is *the larger the discontinuity, the smaller the indication of the received pulse on the CRT.*

Turn ahead to page 4-24.

Incorrect. It is true that bubblers can use both the straight and angle beam techniques but there is no special advantage in using a "bubbler." You will recall that both of these techniques are readily applied to conventional immersion testing.

Now let's take another look at the other selection "no immersion test tank is required." Suppose we have a large specimen that is too large to be placed in an immersion tank, but we need the sensitivity and resolution capabilities that only the immersion technique can produce. A logical choice would be a bubbler because no immersion tank is required. Now wouldn't this be an advantage of the bubbler? Of course.

Turn ahead to page 4-26.

Good. Your analysis is correct. In through-transmission testing, as the size of the discontinuity increases, the indication of the received pulse on the CRT will become smaller. More of the sound wave from the transmitting transducer is reflected by the discontinuity and less is able to get to the receiving transducer.

A special application of immersion testing is the "bubbler" or "squirter" illustrated below.

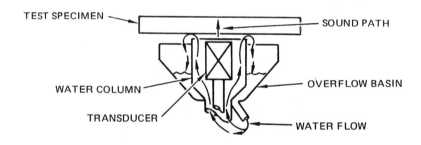

This application is also sometimes referred to as the water column technique. A "bubbler" provides the flexibility of immersion testing without the necessity for large test tanks and elaborate positioning equipment. Both straight and angle beam techniques can be used depending on the bubbler design.

Turn back to page 4-21.

This water-path distance is chosen so that the first multiple of the front surface reflection will not appear until after the back surface reflection has appeared.

Which of the following will be the result if the transducer is placed too close to the test specimen's front surface?

Spurious indication . . . . **Page 4-27**
Loss of back surface reflection . . . . **Page 4-29**

Correct. The fact that no immersion tank is required can be considered an advantage of the bubbler application. The immersion principle can still be used even though the test specimen may be too large for immersion as in conventional immersion testing.

The following illustration shows immersion testing using a straight beam and the CRT indications that will be received.

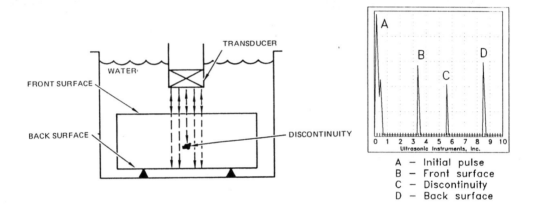

A — Initial pulse
B — Front surface
C — Discontinuity
D — Back surface

When positioning the transducer above the test specimen, a water-path distance is chosen so that the length of time it takes for the sound to travel from the transducer to the surface of the test specimen and back is longer than the length of time it takes for the sound to travel from the front surface of the test article to the back surface and back to the front surface.

Turn back to page 4-25.

Good.　When the transducer is too close to the front surface of the test specimen, the second front surface reflection will appear on the CRT between the first front and back surface reflections.　This first front surface multiple reflection can be misconstrued as the reflection of a discontinuity.

The transducer must be positioned so that it is further from the front surface with respect to the time required for sound travel in water than the time required for the sound beam to travel through the test specimen and be reflected from the back surface.　This is especially important when the test area is gated for automatic recording.

Turn ahead to page 4-31.

Good.   The correct distance between the transducer and the test specimen in this test situation is 1 inch (25.4 mm).

Angle beam testing with immersion techniques is illustrated below.

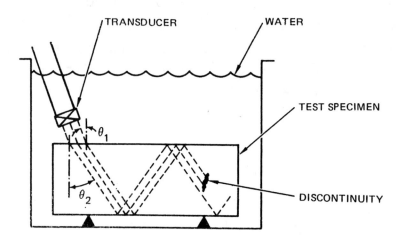

The test setup shown above will produce an indication that differs from that received with straight beam testing due to the angled incidence of the sound beam at the test surface as shown on the page 4-34.

Turn ahead to page 4-34.

Apparently we haven't been too clear in our explanation. We'll try again.

Let's consider for a moment only what is happening between the transducer and the front surface of the test specimen. The ultrasonic pulse is reflected back and forth between the transducer and the front surface of the specimen until all the sound is attenuated. On the CRT, these multiple reflections might appear as shown here.

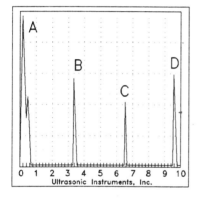

A — Initial pulse
B — Front surface indication
C — First multiple front surface indication
D — Second multiple front surface indication

Now let's consider only what is happening between the transducer and the back surface of the specimen. The reflection from the back surface might cause an indication as shown here.

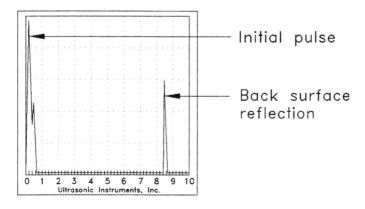

Initial pulse

Back surface reflection

Turn to the next page.

Now, to show everything that might happen we combine the two CRT presentations as shown here.

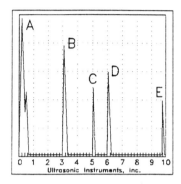

A — Initial pulse
B — Front surface indication
C — First multiple front surface indication
D — Back surface indication
E — Second multiple front surface indication

Notice that the first multiple front surface reflection is appearing ahead of the back surface reflection. This is not desirable since the first multiple front surface reflection could be mistaken for the reflection from a discontinuity.

To move that first multiple front surface reflection so that it appears after the back surface reflection, the water distance has to be increased. We can increase the water distance by moving the transducer further away from the test specimen.

Got it? Good. Now turn back to page 4-27.

The velocity of sound in water is approximately one-fourth the velocity of sound in aluminum or steel. One inch (25.4 mm) of water will appear on the CRT presentation over the same time span as 4 inches (10.2 cm) of steel.

A good rule to remember is that *the distance from the transducer to the test specimen must be at least one quarter of the thickness of the test specimen plus 1/4 inch (6.3 mm)* as illustrated below.

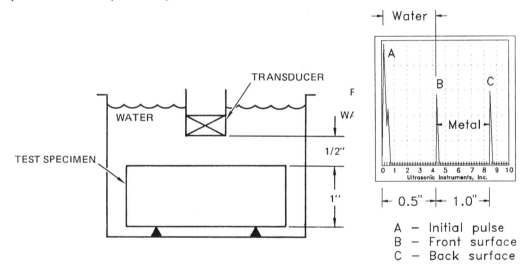

A — Initial pulse
B — Front surface
C — Back surface

Assume you are making a setup to test a flat plate that is *3 inches (76.2 mm)* thick. How much water distance is required between the transducer and top surface of the sheet?

1 inch (25.4 mm) .... **Page 4-28**
1-1/2 inches (38.1 mm) .... **Page 4-32**

No—you must have guessed at the answer by turning to this page. The water distance must be 1/4 of the thickness of the specimen plus 1/4 inch (6.3 mm). The thickness of the specimen is given as 3 inches (76.2 mm).

One-quarter of the thickness is 3/4 inch (19 mm); add 1/4 inch (6.3 mm) and your answer is 1 inch (25.4 mm).

Turn back to page 4-28.

Fine. You remembered the difference between "reflection" and "refraction." In this case the sound is reflected at the test surface at an angle so the majority of the sound beam does not return to the transducer.

Turn ahead to page 4-35.

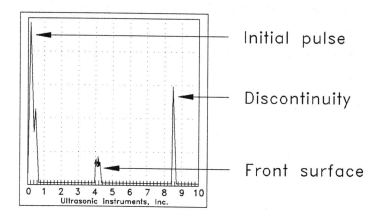

Initial pulse

Discontinuity

Front surface

What is the reason for the low amplitude front surface indication when using angle beam techniques?

Scattered reflection of sound at test surface . . . . **Page 4-33**
Scattered refraction of sound at test surface . . . . **Page 4-36**

Calibration of immersion test equipment, as with contact test equipment, is a check that is made to assure that the test system will provide proper response to signals from artificial discontinuities in test blocks. This operation is performed before each series of ultrasonic tests.

Different calibration procedures are used, depending on the test to be conducted or even on personal preference. Following is a typical calibration procedure. First, examine this setup.

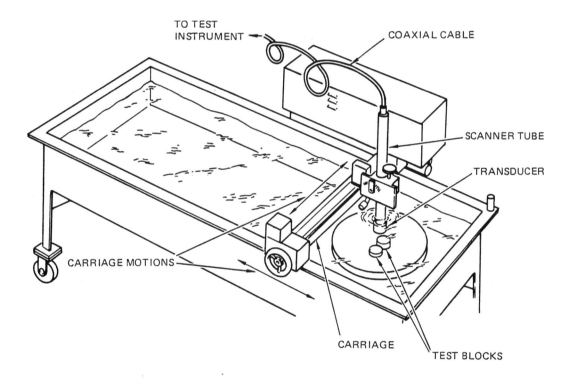

Turn ahead to page 4-37.

Looks as if you were caught napping on this one. Refraction is what occurs *inside the test specimen* when the sound beam is *bent* due to the difference in sound velocity in water and the specimen. In this case the sound is *reflected* at the surface. All of the sound does not return to the transducer due to the angle at which reflection occurs.

Turn back to page 4-33.

- First, two distance amplitude test blocks are selected that are of the same material as that to be tested or of the material prescribed by the test procedure. Each block should contain a 3/64-inch (1.2 mm) flat-bottomed hole, one having a sound-path distance corresponding to the thickness of the material to be tested and the other having a 1/2-inch (12.7 mm) sound-path distance. These are placed in the test tank.

- The transducer is then positioned over the longest block, slightly off-center and normal to the surface (perpendicular). The reflections are observed on the CRT. Water travel distance is adjusted with the manipulator so that the first multiple front surface indication occurs after the first back surface indication. The front surface and first multiple front surface indications can be identified by moving the transducer up and down. As the transducer is moved, the indications will move across the display. The front and back surface indications will maintain the same relationship to each other, while the first multiple front surface indication will change position relative to the front surface indication.

Turn to the next page.

●   Next, the transducer angle is adjusted to obtain a front surface indication on the CRT of maximum height to indicate that the sound beam is striking the surface of the test block squarely. Typical CRT indications are shown in the illustration.

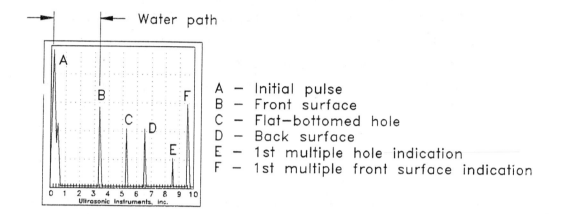

A — Initial pulse
B — Front surface
C — Flat-bottomed hole
D — Back surface
E — 1st multiple hole indication
F — 1st multiple front surface indication

Turn to the next page.

●   The transducer is then moved laterally to a position where the maximum response from the flat-bottomed hole is obtained. The test instrument sensitivity (gain) is then adjusted to produce a full-scale indication from the flat-bottomed hole. The first multiple reflection of the flat-bottomed hole must be at least one-half the height of the first indication. For example, if the measured height of the first indication is 80% FSH, the second indication should be 40% FSH. This relationship is illustrated below.

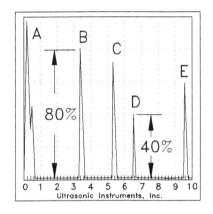

A — Front surface indication
B — Flat—bottomed hole indication
C — Back surface indication
D — 1st multiple hole indication
E — 1st multiple front surface indication

●   Then, without changing instrument adjustment, the transducer is positioned over the second test block containing a sound-path distance of 1/2 inch (12.7 mm) to the flat-bottomed hole. The display should still show the full-scale indication of the flat-bottomed hole and the half-scale indication of the first multiple of the flat-bottomed hole. If the amplitude of these indications is less than those obtained from the block with the longer sound-path distance, increase the instrument sensitivity to obtain this minimum signal strength.

Turn to the next page.

● Last, but not least, the water distance between the transducer and the test block is measured and recorded. This distance must be maintained within plus or minus 1/2 inch (12.7 mm) during testing.

Which of the following statements most nearly describes the reason for selection of the two test blocks in the above procedure?

To check for uniform response over full specimen thickness . . . . **Page 4-42**
The 3/64-inch (1.2 mm) flat-bottomed hole is the smallest to be used for comparison with actual discontinuities . . . **Page 4-44**

It must be remembered that the discontinuity will be directly beneath the transducer only when a straight beam is being used. When the beam is entering the surface at an angle, the amount of refraction must be taken into consideration as we have shown.

Assume now that you have located the discontinuity. You wish to determine if its axis lies at a shallow (parallel) or steep (perpendicular) angle to the surface. Increase the angle of incidence of the beam from 5° to 10° and move the transducer to pick up the strongest indication from the discontinuity.

If the discontinuity indication is decreased, the discontinuity is:

at a steep angle to the surface . . . . **Page 4-45**

at a shallow angle to the surface . . . . **Page 4-46**

You're right. The main reason for selecting one block with 1/2-inch (12.7 mm) sound-path distance from the front surface to the flat-bottomed hole and the other with a sound-path distance that approximates the thickness of the test specimen is to check and adjust the test instrument so that the response is uniform over the full range of test specimen thickness.

Now, let's assume that we are manually checking a specimen and a discontinuity indication appears on the CRT. How can the position of the discontinuity in the specimen be determined?

If a straight beam is being used, the discontinuity will be directly below the transducer. If an angle beam is being used, we have a problem—the refraction of the sound beam has to be taken into consideration. Here's how we can find the physical location of a discontinuity when the beam hits the surface at an angle. First examine this diagram.

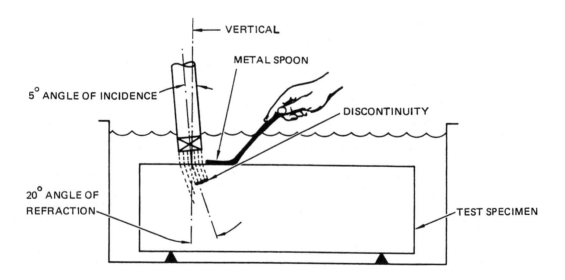

Turn to the next page.

CRT indications during such a test might look like this.

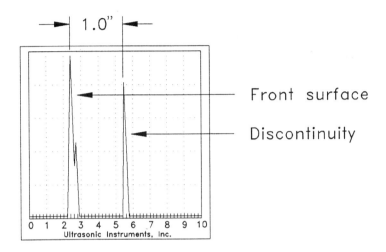

From the previous illustration, we know that the discontinuity is about 1 inch (25.4 mm) below the test surface along an angle of 20° from where the sound beam strikes the surface. What we don't know is exactly where the sound beam strikes the surface.

The point at which the sound beam strikes the surface can be determined by placing a straight-edged piece of metal (metal spoon in the illustration) on the surface of the specimen and moving it toward the area where the sound is entering the test surface. As soon as the leading edge of the metal enters the sound beam, an indication will appear on the CRT. This point is marked on the test surface. The same check is then performed from the other three sides of the beam. This procedure locates the area in which the sound beam *enters* the specimen.

Turn back to page 4-41.

Your answer is not the best of the two available. It is true that a 3/64-inch (1.2 mm) flat-bottomed hole may be the smallest that will be used for comparison with actual discontinuities, but the main reason for selecting the two blocks (one block with a sound-path distance the same as the specimen and the other 1/2 inch or 12.7 mm from the test surface) is so that the instrument may be adjusted to obtain *uniform response* over the full specimen thickness.

Turn back to page 4-42.

Perhaps you don't understand the situation we've just described. The illustration below is a diagram of the situation. We are assuming here that the axis of the discontinuity is at a shallow angle to the surface.

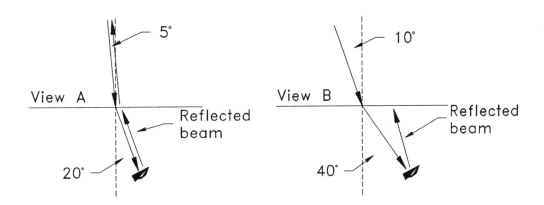

View A shows the axis of the discontinuity lying approximately perpendicular to the refracted angle of 20°. This situation results in a strong signal from the discontinuity.

In View B we have changed the angle of incidence to 10° and have relocated the transducer to the point where we received the strongest indication of the discontinuity. Since the discontinuity is no longer perpendicular to the angle of refraction, most of the beam is reflected away from the transducer.

Now can you see that if the indication decreases when we go from the first situation to the second, the axis of the discontinuity is at a shallow angle?

Turn to the next page.

Good. If the angle of sound beam incidence is increased and the resultant indication of the discontinuity on the CRT decreases, the discontinuity lies at a shallow angle to the test surface. The added angulation causes more of the sound beam to be reflected off the discontinuity away from the transducer.

Before going on to the application of immersion testing, we should consider the wave modes that can be used in immersion testing.

Here, unlike contact testing, surface wave testing would not be possible due to the liquid bath. By using the angle beam technique, sound can be propagated in the specimen in both the longitudinal and shear wave modes, depending on the test conditions and requirements.

From what you've learned about the different wave modes and their characteristics, which of the following waves *cannot* be used in immersion testing?

Plate waves . . . . **Page 4-47**
Surface waves . . . . **Page 4-48**

Your answer is incorrect. Plate waves *can* be produced in thin sheets using conventional immersion techniques, normally using a two-transducer testing technique. It is *surface waves* that cannot be produced in immersion testing.

Recall what you've learned about surface waves. You'll remember that a surface wave can be dampened out by water, grease, your finger, or just about anything placed in its path on the surface of a test specimen. Therefore, we find that in immersion testing these waves are dampened so soon after the start of propagation that it is impossible to use them for test purposes.

Turn to page 4-48.

Good. You remembered that a surface wave will not propagate in water. Water causes a dampening effect and a useful reflection cannot be obtained. Plate waves, on the other hand, can be produced in thin sheets and used in immersion testing.

Now for a review on what you've learned about immersion testing.

Turn to the next page.

CHAPTER REVIEW

1. In immersion testing, the principal function of water is its use as a:

    A.   couplant.
    B.   detergent.
    C.   rust inhibitor.
    D.   softener.

2. One of the main advantages of immersion testing is the use of _____ frequencies so that smaller discontinuities can be detected.

    A.   low
    B.   high

3. The device used to adjust the angle of the transducer so that the sound beam can be transmitted into a test specimen at an angle is the:

    A.   carriage.
    B.   angulator.
    C.   manipulator.
    D.   oscillator.

____   4.   The _____ provides a mounting for the transducer and is raised or lowered to change the water distance between the transducer and test specimen.

A.   carriage
B.   manipulator
C.   oscillator
D.   scanner tube

____   5.   Given a choice of a 5-MHz, 10-MHz, 15-MHz or 20-MHz transducer, the _____-MHz transducer should be chosen for the best resolution of small discontinuities.

A.   5
B.   10
C.   15
D.   20

____   6.   When using a focused transducer, you can normally expect to receive _____ back surface reflection(s).

A.   no
B.   a large
C.   multiple
D.   three

7.	A special application of immersion testing in which an immersion tank is not required is referred to as the _____ technique.

	A.	bubbler
	B.	squirter
	C.	water column
	D.	All of the above.

8.	When a transducer is placed too close to the front surface of a test specimen, the second front surface reflection will appear _____ the back surface reflection on the CRT.

	A.	on top of
	B.	after
	C.	before
	D.	to be masked by

9.	The distance from the transducer to the test specimen should be at least equal to _____ of the thickness of the specimen plus _____.

	A.	1/2, 1/2 inch (12.7 mm, 12.7 mm)
	B.	1/4, 1/4 inch (6.3 mm, 6.3 mm)
	C.	1, 1/4 inch (25.4 mm, 6.3 mm)
	D.	1/2, 1 inch (12.7 mm, 25.4 mm)

10.   _____ is the name given to a check by the operator to assure that the test system will provide proper response to reflections from artificial reflectors in test blocks.

    A.   Oscillation
    B.   Immersion
    C.   Calibration
    D.   Tip diffraction

11.   In immersion testing, a flat _____ may be used to determine the area in which the ultrasonic beam enters the test specimen.

    A.   horse shoe
    B.   metal spoon
    C.   manipulator
    D.   immersion tank

12.   Assume that you receive an 80% FSH front surface reflection when testing with the sound beam striking the surface at a 90° angle (perpendicular). When the transducer angle is changed to 20°, the front surface indication will become:

    A.   smaller.
    B.   larger.
    C.   much wider.
    D.   inverted.

_____   13.   With the exception of _____ waves, all wave modes
                can be produced in test specimens with conventional
                immersion testing techniques.

                A.   plate
                B.   shear
                C.   Lamb
                D.   surface

Turn to the next page for answers to these review questions.

ANSWERS TO REVIEW QUESTIONS
FOR CHAPTER 4

Question & Answer		Reference Page(s)
1.	A	4-2
2.	B	4-14
3.	C	4-3
4.	D	4-9
5.	D	4-14
6.	A	4-18
7.	D	4-21, 4-24
8.	C	4-25, 4-27
9.	B	4-31
10.	C	4-35
11.	B	4-43
12.	A	4-45
13.	D	4-46, 4-47

Turn to the next page and begin Chapter 5.

CHAPTER 5

APPLICATION OF IMMERSION TESTING

Before going into a few of the typical applications of immersion testing, let's consider how we can determine if the discontinuities found will be cause for rejection of the specimen.

The test procedure will tell us that discontinuities providing a reflection greater than that provided by an artificial reflector of certain dimensions will be cause for rejection. Or, in other cases, the test procedure will tell us that if the discontinuities are of certain size and are closely spaced, the specimen shall be rejected.

One approach to evaluating discontinuities is as follows:

- Select a test block with a artificial reflector as specified in the test procedure that has a sound-path distance very nearly equal to the sound path of the discontinuity.
- Position the transducer above the test block with the same water distance as used in testing the specimen.
- Obtain a discontinuity indication from the artificial reflector or flat-bottomed hole in the test block.
- Compare the overall response of any discontinuity indication to that of the reflector at a similar sound-path distance.
- The discontinuity may be rejectable if the conditions, such as material thickness, material properties, service conditions, etc., warrant a concern for the use or continued use of the test article.

Turn to the next page.

Many factors play a role in the acceptance or rejection of a component based on nondestructive tests. Various governing bodies have issued codes that evaluate the discontinuity characteristics and compare these to failure analysis histograms.

Assume that you have a 50% FSH indication from both a discontinuity and a flat-bottomed hole at a similar sound-path distance in the material.

Which is the larger of the two?

The flat-bottomed hole .... **Page 5-4**
The discontinuity .... **Page 5-6**

Contoured surfaces can be easily tested with immersion techniques. Some ultrasonic testing installations have facilities for automatic scanning of complex shapes with the automatic equipment driven by a micro (or personal) computer to match the contour of the specimen. The computer program assures that the water distance and transducer angulation is automatically adjusted to match the change in test surface contour.

Turn ahead to page 5-8.

Did you forget? Any time you receive reflections that are of equal amplitude from a discontinuity and a flat-bottomed hole, you always judge the discontinuity to be the larger.

A flat-bottomed hole has a smooth reflecting surface and there will be little scattering of the sound beam. The majority of the sound will be returned to the transducer for display on the CRT.

On the other hand, the reflecting surface of discontinuities are usually rougher than that of a flat-bottomed hole. Some of the sound beam will scatter and will not be returned to the transducer, and the resulting indication will be smaller.

Turn ahead to page 5-6.

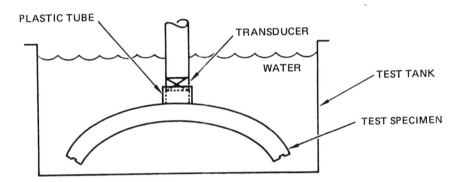

The plastic tube, illustrated again above, provides proper spacing between the transducer and the test specimen and is properly shaped to follow the contour of the specimen.

Which of the following properties of the tube describes the effects on the sound beam?

Contains and directs the sound beam . . . . **Page 5-7**
Adds acoustic impedance . . . . **Page 5-9**

Excellent. You remembered that a discontinuity can always be considered to be the larger when equal magnitude indications are received from a discontinuity and a flat-bottomed hole at the same sound-path distance in the material. The test procedure takes this fact into account when it specifies a standard for comparison.

Turn back to page 5-3.

Correct. In addition to the mechanical job of maintaining proper spacing between the transducer and the specimen and adjusting to the contour of the specimen, the plastic tube *contains and directs the sound beam.*

Now let's discuss the testing of cylindrically-shaped specimens. First, we will consider the testing of ring forgings with shear waves.

The ring forging is positioned with its longitudinal axis in a vertical direction in the tank so as to permit rotation of the forging as shown below. When shear wave techniques are to be used, a notch is cut into the radial thickness of the forging and the test instrument calibrated to reflections from the notch.

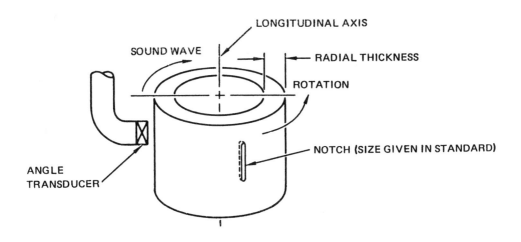

A right-angle transducer is used to project an angle beam into the rotating forging with the beam angled to enter the specimen in the direction opposite to the direction of rotation. The test instrument sensitivity is adjusted to obtain a maximum indication on the CRT from the notch. During the test on the forging, any discontinuity indications exceeding the indication from the notch will be cause for rejection.

Turn ahead to page 5-10.

Hand-controlled scanning of contoured surfaces can be accomplished through the use of a hollow plastic extension tube on the end of the transducer. The tube is placed in contact with the test surface to maintain proper distance between the transducer and the specimen at all times. Where the specimen has a constant curvature similar to that shown in the following illustration, the plastic tube is shaped to fit the contour of the specimen to maintain normal incidence of the sound beam.

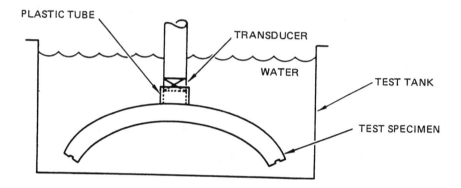

Turn back to page 5-5.

Don't forget—the tube is hollow. The plastic tube does not add acoustic impedance to affect the sound beam. Actually, any errant sound beam in the column of water within the tube will reflect back into the column of water. In this application, the plastic tube "contains and directs" the sound beam.

Turn back to page 5-7.

The ring is scanned from top to bottom, moving the transducer successively downward after each revolution of the ring.

Assume there exists a discontinuity in the ring forging. Which of the following indications will appear on the CRT?

Small front and back surface and discontinuity reflections . . . . **Page 5-12**
Small front surface and discontinuity reflections . . . . **Page 5-14**

During testing, the forging is rotated while the transducer is held in a position perpendicular to the surface. Discontinuity indications will be conventionally displayed on the CRT between the front and back surface indications.

The forging will normally be considered defective if discontinuity indications exceed a percentage of the back surface indication as specified in the test procedure.

Select the best completion for the following statement. The process of adjusting a test instrument to provide a controlled response under simulated test conditions is known as:

a factory (or manufacturer's) calibration . . . . **Page 5-13**
a system calibration . . . . **Page 5-16**

Your answer is partially correct. In the test situation under consideration, the sound beam is striking a curved surface at an angle. In the question we assumed there was a discontinuity, so the following illustration portrays what is observed on the CRT.

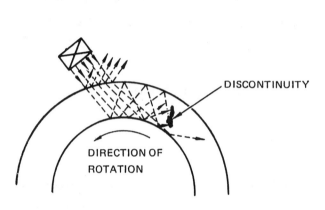

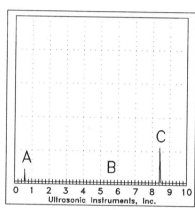

A — Front surface
B — Back surface
C — Discontinuity

True, the front surface indication will be small because a lot (but not all) of the sound beam will be reflected away from the transducer.

Because the sonic beam strikes the back surface of the specimen at an even greater incident angle, even less of the beam will be reflected back to the transducer.

The size of the discontinuity indication depends, of course, upon the size of the discontinuity, its reflective surface, and its orientation within the part.

Turn ahead to page 5-14.

No—a factory calibration, or manufacturer's calibration, is the periodic *adjustment of an instrument in a laboratory under controlled conditions with the use of precise standards.* This process checks the performance of all electronic circuits as well as the capability of the instrument to provide indications from calibrated reference blocks similar to the test blocks used for system calibration.

System calibration is adjustment of a test instrument to provide a controlled response under simulated test conditions.

Turn ahead to page 5-16.

Good. This question is an adaptation of what you studied previously about the effects of an angle beam striking a curved surface. We will receive only a small front surface reflection and a reflection from the discontinuity.

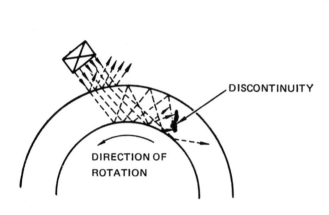

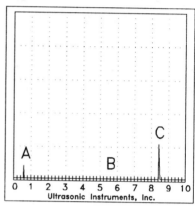

A — Front surface
B — Back surface
C — Discontinuity

Straight beam testing can also be applied to testing ring forgings. In this case, the instrument is calibrated by projecting the sound beam perpendicular to the surface. Instrument sensitivity is adjusted so that the back surface indication is at least 75% FSH on the CRT screen. A notch is not used in this case.

Turn back to page 5-11.

Your answer is incorrect. The initial scanning pass with the transducer in the center of the specimen will result in longitudinal waves. As the transducer moves further from the center, the refracted angle will first cause longitudinal and shear waves to exist in the specimen; then as it moves further away from the center, only shear waves will be produced. Scanning ceases at the point where shear wave refraction reaches 90° (second critical angle), the angle at which surface waves are produced. Remember, surface waves are dampened out by water couplant in immersion testing and cannot exist. Therefore, we can say that only *longitudinal and shear waves* will exist in the test specimen as scanning progresses from the center of the test specimen outward.

Turn ahead to page 5-18.

Very good.   The process of *adjusting a test instrument to provide a controlled response under simulated test conditions* is known as *calibrating the test system.*

Round bar stock, tubing, and curved sections of forgings may be tested using "off-center" scanning techniques. In this technique, the transducer is positioned parallel to the vertical diameter of the test specimen but is displaced to one side of the center as shown in the illustration below (Point B). With the probe off-center, the test surface is at an angle other than normal to the sound beam and refraction occurs.

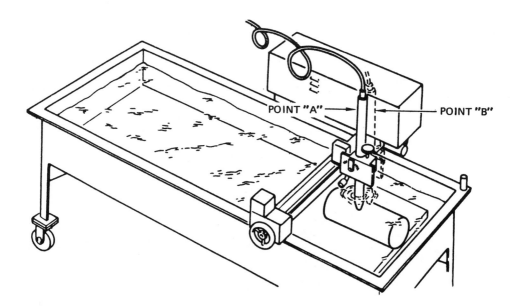

Turn to the next page.

Scanning commences from the center, Point A in the proceeding figure, where the refracted angle is zero. The scanning pass is completed by moving the transducer in one direction until a point is reached where the shear wave mode is refracted 90° (second critical angle). This scanning technique will assure that radial discontinuities will be intersected at right angles to the face of the discontinuity so the sound will be reflected in the proper direction for display on the CRT.

When scanning with the above technique, which of the following wave modes will exist in the test specimen?

Shear and surface waves . . . . **Page 5-15**
Longitudinal and shear waves . . . . **Page 5-18**

Right. Longitudinal and shear waves will exist in the test specimen as scanning progresses from the center outward, depending upon the angle of incidence at the test surface.

Immersion testing of pipe and tubing can be accomplished on a production line basis using either conventional techniques with the transducer immersed in water or by use of a "bubbler" where the sound beam is projected through a water column.

Turn to the next page.

Typical ultrasonic indications that may be obtained on a CRT while testing
specimens with different wall thicknesses are shown below. View A shows
the behavior of the sound beam when testing thin-walled tubing. Much of
the sound is reflected from the surface, and sound which enters the
specimen is trapped in the tube wall and travels around the circumference
until it strikes a discontinuity that causes a reflection. When no
discontinuities are present, only a very small front surface indication will be
received.

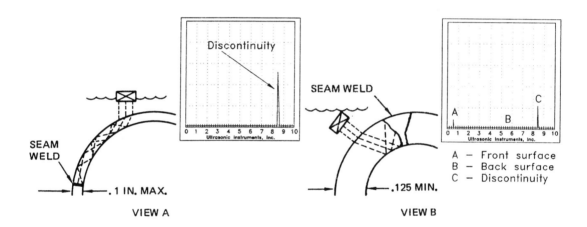

View B shows the sound beam entering a thicker-walled tube. Again, the
sound is trapped in the tube wall, but different reflections may occur due
to the greater wall thickness. In tubes larger than about 0.125-inch (3.2
mm) wall thickness, small front and back surface reflections may occur;
discontinuity indications will cause a much larger indication and are readily
detected.

**The only difference in the above test setups and conditions that cause
different indications is the:**

tube wall thickness .... **Page 5-21**

angle of sound beam incidence .... **Page 5-23**

If the weld seam contains no discontinuities, no indication will appear on the CRT; however, if there is a discontinuity, an indication will appear that is proportional in amplitude to the reflectivity and orientation of the discontinuity's surface. The test procedure will dictate what the acceptance limits are.

The position of this indication will not change and will be determined by the constant distance between the transducer and welded seam. It is also possible to equip the testing system with a marking device that will automatically mark the tube when a discontinuity indication is received. Process control feedback devices may cause a defective tube or pipe to be sorted or rerouted for further analysis.

In this type of testing only the weld area is inspected. What feature of the test instrument will prevent the recording of unwanted discontinuity reflections?

Gate . . . . **Page 5-22**
Sweep delay . . . . **Page 5-24**

That is correct. The only thing that causes the difference in the two CRT indications is the *thickness of the tube walls*.

Now let's look at a technique used in high-speed scanning of welds in tubing. After welding, tubing is passed through holes in the ends of an ultrasonic immersion tank; the holes are so designed that water is retained in the tank.

The transducer is fastened to a holder that rides on the surface of the tubing as shown in the following illustration. The seam in the tube always occupies the same position with relation to the transducer. The sound beam strikes the surface of the tube at an angle producing a sound wave in the tube wall that travels around the circumference and strikes the welded seam at right angles.

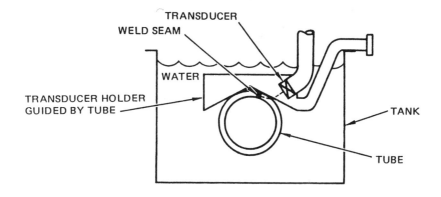

Turn back to page 5-20.

That's right. An electronic gate on the test system can be used so that only those reflections that occur in the weld area will be *recorded*. Discontinuity reflections from other areas around the circumference of the tube can be seen on the face of the CRT but will not be recorded since only the weld area will be gated.

A variation of the immersion technique in testing of tubing using a "bubbler" is illustrated below. Tubes are drawn across the transducer which is positioned to allow sound energy to enter the tube wall at a point 90° from the welded area.

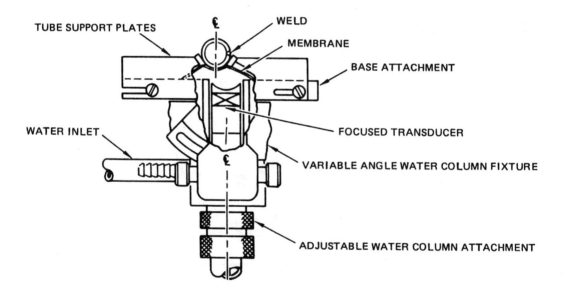

Turn ahead to page 5-25.

Incorrect. The only difference between the two examples is the *thickness* of the tube wall. In this case, we are considering that the same angle of incidence is used. If the angle of incidence is changed, there will be different reflections in each of the specimens; however, that factor is not to be taken into consideration in these examples.

Turn back to page 5-21.

The question asked what feature of the test instrument will prevent the recording of unwanted discontinuity reflections. You chose "sweep delay." This is not correct.

The sweep delay feature of the instrument allows us to delay the start of the sweep on the CRT to allow "erasing" the water distance from the face of the CRT. We will still see all indications that are due to reflections from discontinuities around the circumference of the tube.

If we want to *record* only the discontinuities that the sound beam detects in the weld area, we use the electronic gate. Discontinuities occurring outside the gated area will cause reflections that we can see on the face of the CRT but, due to the gate, only indications from discontinuities within the gated area will be recorded.

Turn back to page 5-22.

Discontinuity indications will occur under the same conditions as those described when the transducer and tube are immersed in water. Automatic marking, recording and/or process feedback control devices may also be used with this system to designate areas of the tube that contain discontinuities or to reroute defective tubes.

What sort of calibrating device is used for comparison with discontinuities detected in tubing when tested by the above technique?

Area amplitude test blocks . . . . **Page 5-27**
Notches in good section of tubing . . . . **Page 5-30**

Your answer is wrong. Mode conversion to transform the wave from longitudinal to shear does not occur until the sound beam strikes the entry surface of the test specimen. At that point it is transformed into shear waves. The sound wave travels in the shear mode while in the specimen and is converted to the longitudinal mode at the interface before returning to the transducer for display on the CRT.

Turn ahead to page 5-28.

By turning to this page you indicate that you think that area amplitude test blocks are used for calibrating the instrument for comparison with discontinuity indications from tubing. This is not correct.

Remember what you learned about ultrasonic testing of tubing in the chapters on contact testing? You learned that tubing *standards are prepared by cutting notches in the inner and outer diameter of the tube.* Reflections from these notches are the standards against which reflections from discontinuities are compared.

The size of the notches is not important at this time. This information will be set forth in the test procedures.

Turn ahead to page 5-30.

Right. The wave mode is longitudinal during the time the sound beam is traveling through the water between the transducer and the test surface.

The area of bonding between two materials can be tested ultrasonically with good results. The following illustration shows a technique that is used with automatic scanning and recording equipment. A focused transducer with the focal zone at the area of the bond is used to test the area between the two materials. Results are printed out in B-scan, C-scan, or D-scan on a multicolored printer or plotter.

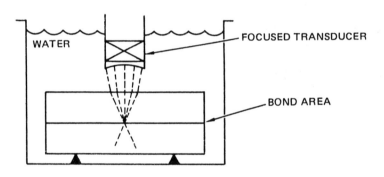

Assume that you are to conduct a test of bonding. Transducers of 10 MHz and 20 MHz are available for use.

Which should you select for the best resolution of lack of bond discontinuities?

10 MHz .... **Page 5-32**
20 MHz .... **Page 5-34**

Good. You are so right. View A indicates that the sound beam has penetrated the bond area. In the areas where there is lack of bond (View C), the sound beam is principally reflected and does not penetrate the interface.

Turn ahead to page 5-35 for a short review of the material contained in this chapter.

Very good. Indications as a result of reflections from notches in a good section of tubing are used as standards to which reflections from discontinuities are compared.

The use of immersion testing techniques to test butt welds in heavy plate is illustrated below.

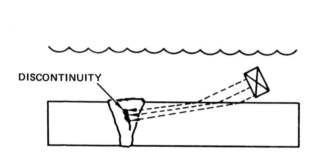

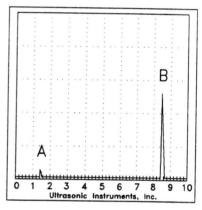

A — Front surface
B — Discontinuity

When the sound beam enters the test surface at an angle, refraction will occur in the test specimen. Small changes in the angle of incidence will cause much larger changes in the refracted angle due to the difference of sound velocity in water and metal. Usually it is desirable in weld testing to generate shear waves in the test specimen. To generate shear waves, the transducer is tilted to an angle of incidence between 15° and 33°.

Turn to the next page.

In shear wave testing, a small poorly-defined reflection will be returned from the surface while a strong reflection will be returned from vertical fissures or cracks in the test specimen.

If the transducer is moved horizontally toward the weld, the discontinuity indication will move toward the front surface indication because the path of the sound wave in the specimen is made shorter.

Which of the following wave modes best describes the particle motion while the sound beam is traveling through the water?

Shear waves .... **Page 5-26**
Longitudinal waves .... **Page 5-28**

Your selection will not give you the best resolution of very small discontinuities. The best choice would be 20 MHz, since the wavelength will be shorter at the higher frequency. One of the basic rules of ultrasonics is that *the shorter the wavelength, the smaller the discontinuity that can be detected*.

Turn ahead to page 5-34.

View A indicates the bonding is good. Right? This means that the sound beam has penetrated through the majority of the bonded area and was not reflected. This C-scan is at the depth of the interface and represents a good bond. Note the contrast to View C which reflects at the bond interface location or depth. In this case your selection of an answer should have been "an acceptable bond interface."

Turn back to page 5-29.

Excellent. The higher frequency will give the best resolution of the very small discontinuities such as you are looking for in checking the bonding quality between two materials.

Metal-to-honeycomb bonding, commonly known as a "honeycomb bond," can likewise be successfully tested with the immersion testing technique. The degree of bonding, as well as the lack of bond, can be detected since the degree of bonding is directly related to the acoustic impedance mismatch at the interface between the two materials.

The amount of sound energy that is reflected from or transmitted through the interface is directly related to the degree of bonding. Variations in the quality of the bond will be shown as alterations in the presence and/or amplitude of reflected signals. Illustrated below are C-scans of a typical honeycomb bond for an aircraft wing structure.

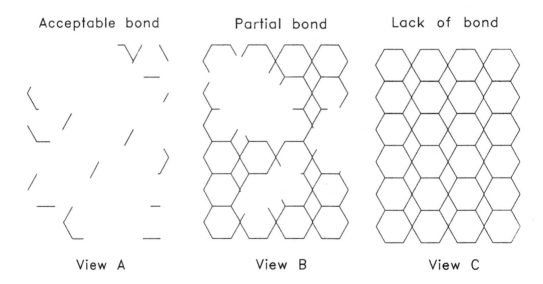

Acceptable bond   Partial bond   Lack of bond

View A   View B   View C

Which of the following conditions does View A above indicate?

An acceptable bond interface . . . . **Page 5-29**
A lack of bonding at the interface . . . . **Page 5-33**

CHAPTER REVIEW

_____ 1. When comparing the amplitude of a discontinuity indication with that of an equal magnitude indication from a flat-bottomed hole, the discontinuity can always be considered to be:

    A. the same size.
    B. smaller.
    C. longer.
    D. larger.

_____ 2. Hand scanning of contoured surfaces using immersion techniques may require the use of a plastic extension tube on the end of the transducer. The tube is necessary to assure that the _____ is the same at all test points.

    A. tube length
    B. test article
    C. transducer shape
    D. water distance

_____ 3. Particle motion when the sound beam is traveling through water between the transducer and test specimen is always in the _____ mode.

    A. surface
    B. plate
    C. longitudinal
    D. shear

_____ 4. Assume you are testing a ring forging using an angle beam. Will you normally expect to receive a reflection from the back surface?

A. Yes
B. No

_____ 5. Angle beam immersion testing, like angle beam contact testing, requires the use of _____ to evaluate discontinuities in ring forgings, piping, and tubing.

A.   propagation devices
B.   flattened standards
C.   reference notches
D.   code cases

_____ 6. When testing a ring forging using a straight beam technique, the forging is considered defective if any discontinuity indication exceeds a specified percentage of the _____ reflection as given in the test procedure.

A.   back surface
B.   front surface
C.   left edge
D.   bottom half

_____ 7. Different CRT indications can be expected when testing tubing with thin walls than those obtained from tubing with thick walls. Assume that thin-walled tubing is being tested with an angle beam. Will you expect to see a reflection from the back surface?

A. Yes
B. No

_____ 8. During production-line testing of welds in tubing, the test system is adjusted so that reflections from the weld area are the only ones that will cause a process feedback device to be actuated. The _____ circuit in the system provides this feature.

A. pulser
B. receiver
C. gating
D. clock

_____ 9. A small poorly-defined reflection may be returned from the entry surface of a test specimen when using _____ beam immersion methods.

A. angle
B. through
C. straight
D. convoluted

_____ 10. Assume a test of bonding between two materials is to be made. A choice of 5-MHz, 10-MHz, 15-MHz, and 20-MHz transducers is available. The best resolution of lack of bond discontinuities will be obtained if the _____-MHz transducer is used.

A.   20
B.   15
C.   10
D.   5

_____ 11. When pulse-echo testing bonding between two materials, a strong CRT indication will be received from the bond area when the bond is:

A.   good.
B.   bad.
C.   vertical.
D.   interactive.

Turn to the next page.

Turn to the next page for answers to these review questions.

ANSWERS TO REVIEW QUESTIONS
FOR CHAPTER 5

Question & Answer		Reference Page(s)
1.	D	5-6
2.	D	5-8
3.	C	5-28
4.	B	5-14
5.	C	5-30
6.	A	5-11
7.	B	5-19
8.	C	5-22
9.	A	5-30
10.	A	5-34
11.	B	5-34

Turn to the next page and begin Chapter 6.

CHAPTER 6

NONRELEVANT INDICATIONS

So far in this study of ultrasonic testing we have considered the techniques that are used in testing materials of various shapes and composition. You have also learned what may be expected in the way of indications when discontinuities are encountered in test specimens. In practice, the indications are not as simple as may have been suggested. Many indications are caused by secondary influences from the test system and the test specimen. You need to know of the existence of these, what they look like, and when to disregard them in evaluating the results of ultrasonic tests.

The indications that may be caused by secondary influences are divided into seven classes as follows:

- Electrical interference
- Interference from the transducer
- Interference from the surface of the test specimen
- Interference caused by refraction of the sound beam
- Interference caused by the shape of the test specimen
- Interference caused by material structure
- Accidental interference

The first two classes are caused by malfunctions in the test system—the remainder are inherent in the ultrasonic testing method. The type of indications that may be expected from each of the many possible "nonrelevant indications" will be explained and illustrated on the succeeding pages.

Turn to the next page.

False indications resulting from electrical interference can be due to the effects of noise, a faulty power supply, or sonic reverberations in the test specimen.

Noise can be recognized as a vertical broadening of the baseline or indications that randomly "walk" across the display. This type of noise can be caused by poor electrical contact in the plugs and receptacles that interconnect the transducer and the test instrument, poor electrical contact between the coaxial cable and terminating plugs, or poor electrical contacts within the test instrument.

The indication from noise effects is much the same as the noise that can result from test specimens with relatively coarse grain structures. You learned that this type of noise can be eliminated on instruments with a REJECT control by suppressing unwanted low amplitude indications on the baseline. If the noise indication is caused by electrical interference, use of the REJECT control will have no effect in eliminating the noise.

Noise conditions that are due to poor electrical contact in connections exterior to the test instrument case can usually be corrected by cleaning the electrical plug and receptacles. Electrical noise effects are similar to noise that can be caused by the test specimens.

When noise indications are received, your first step in isolating and correcting the cause of the noise should be to:

determine if it is caused by test system or specimen . . . . Page 6-4
check and clean the electrical plugs and receptacles . . . . Page 6-6

Sorry, but you are wrong. Electrical interference may be caused by the ultrasonic test equipment. If the equipment is defective, many of the faults can be corrected by the operator or the operator can isolate the trouble to determine that it is definitely in the test instrument.

Most importantly these nonrelevant indications will interfere or at least complicate the evaluation process.

Turn ahead to page 6-5.

That's right. When you receive noise effects on the CRT, first determine if the source is the specimen or the test system. If the instrument is so equipped, operate the REJECT control to suppress the noise. If the cause of the noise is in the specimen, the noise indication will disappear; if the cause of the noise is the test system, the noise indication will remain. If the instrument does not have reject capability, lift the transducer from the test specimen. The noise indication will disappear if it is caused by the specimen but will remain if it is a result of the test system.

An apparent discontinuity indication that is moving ("walking") in a horizontal plane along the baseline is often caused by the main electrical power supply, probably due to the use of other industrial equipment on the same power line. This moving indication can be distinguished from a discontinuity since it is irregular and not synchronized with the time base.

Select the best completion for the following statement. The first step in isolating the cause of a moving nonrelevant indication trace should be to:

return it to the manufacturer .... **Page 6-7**
connect the instrument to a different power circuit ...... **Page 6-9**

Correct. The effects of electrical interference can be assessed and often controlled by the ultrasonic operator. These indications serve to complicate the evaluation process.

The next, and last, nonrelevant indication that results from a malfunction in the testing system is due to a defective search unit. A specific type of unwanted indication is usually characterized by a prolonged ringing which widens the initial pulse as shown in the illustration below. View A shows the front surface indication that should be expected from a good transducer; View B shows the type of indication that may result if the crystal should happen to become loose in the search unit. The prolonged ringing effect may result in very little capability of the test system to detect discontinuities.

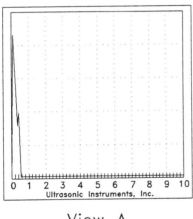
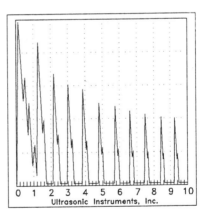

View A   View B

What is the main advantage of a narrow initial pulse?

Better near surface resolution . . . . **Page 6-8**
Better penetrating power . . . . **Page 6-10**

You have decided to check and clean the electrical connections. What if the noise is caused by the test specimen? If so, you might be going to a lot of trouble for nothing.

First, you should determine if the noise is coming from the specimen or if the noise is caused by the test instrument. The cause of the noise can be isolated in one of two ways:

●   If the instrument has a REJECT control, adjust it and if the noise disappears, the test system is operating satisfactorily.

●   If there is no REJECT control, lift the transducer off the test specimen. The noise will disappear if the test system is not defective.

Once the trouble is isolated to the test system, proceed to check and clean the electrical plugs and receptacles.

Turn back to page 6-4.

No—the *most practical first step* to be taken if you encounter a moving indication will be to disconnect the test instrument and *try it out on a different electrical power circuit*. If the problem is caused by industrial equipment that is connected to the first circuit, the indication will disappear when connection is made to a different circuit. If the test system is defective, the moving indication will remain regardless of which electrical circuit is used. If it is determined that the problem is in the instrument, the trouble can normally be isolated to a component in the instrument, although that is not the function of the operator.

Turn ahead to page 6-9.

You're correct. The main advantage of a narrow pulse, and therefore a narrow initial pulse, is detection of discontinuities that lie close to the surface of the test specimen.

During angle beam contact testing using wedges, a certain amount of unwanted reflections are received from the wedge. Reflections within a typical wedge are illustrated below.

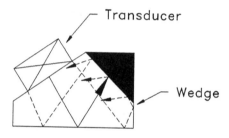

Ordinarily, a portion of the energy from the transducer is reflected away from the transducer at the interface between the wedge and the test specimen. A small amount of this reflected energy may return to the transducer and be displayed. The use of properly-shaped wedges causes a maximum amount of sound attenuation so that the amount actually displayed immediately following the initial pulse is negligible, as illustrated.

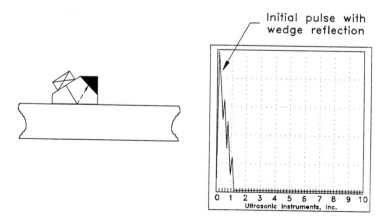

Turn ahead to page 6-11.

Right. The first step in isolating the source of electrical interference that results in a moving indication is to determine whether or not the trouble is in the main electrical power source. If connection to a different electrical circuit has no effect on the indication, then the test system/instrument can be checked and repaired.

Another cause of electrical interference is "wrap around" (reverberation) in the test specimen. Wrap around occurs when the frequency of the pulses emitted by the pulser, or repetition rate, is so frequent that the first pulse does not have time to fully attenuate before the second pulse is initiated. The result will be an apparent discontinuity indication. Decreasing the repetition rate should eliminate the problem.

Interference caused by electrical conditions will interfere with proper evaluation of reflections from discontinuities. The effects of this interference can be assessed by the ultrasonic operator.

False . . . . **Page 6-3**
True . . . . **Page 6-5**

Sorry. Your answer is not correct. Penetrating power is proportional to the amount of energy in the transmitted beam. There is more power in a longer pulse than in a short one.

Remember. A *short pulse* will provide better resolution of discontinuities that lie close to the surface of the test specimen.

Turn back to page 6-8.

The disturbance due to reflections in the wedge can be identified easily by the ultrasonic operator. When the transducer with a plexiglass wedge is lifted off the test specimen, this unwanted indication will usually still be present. One can also finger damp the front of the wedge to reduce and identify this indication.

What can you do to eliminate unwanted reflections from the angle beam wedge?

Add art gum (putty) to the front of the wedge . . . . **Page 6-13**
Experiment with different angles of incidence . . . . **Page 6-14**

Very good. It will definitely be possible to locate discontinuities in the presence of these unwanted surface wave indications. Once the indication is identified as coming from the edge of the specimen, you can disregard it and look for discontinuities within the specimen.

You will recall that surface waves may be used to detect surface cracks in test specimens. Not all reflections that are received from these unwanted surface waves are spurious indications. Some will reveal actual discontinuities.

Assume that you are using angle beam techniques to test a specimen with shear waves. A small surface wave component will be generated as shown in the illustration below. A surface crack may cause a reflection and the display of an indication on the CRT.

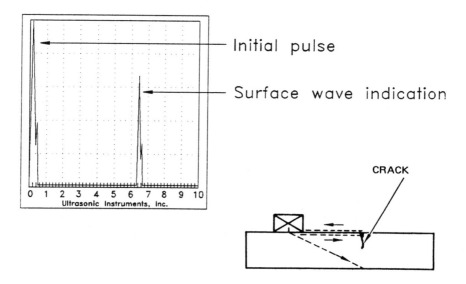

Turn ahead to page 6-17.

That is correct. You could use art gum or a similar putty on the front or top of the wedge to minimize the reflections from the wedge. However, if these indications are occurring between the probe and the surface of the specimen, the operator can do very little. These reflections are inherent to the angle beam method of contact testing. Once it is understood that they will be present to some degree, there will be no difficulty in distinguishing these reflections from actual discontinuity reflections.

Surface waves generated during straight beam (or angle beam) testing can also cause unwanted nonrelevant indications when they are reflected from the edge of a test specimen as illustrated.

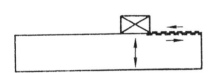

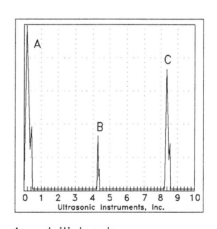

Ultrasonic Instruments, Inc.

A — Initial pulse
B — Surface wave reflection
C — Back surface reflection

Turn ahead to page 6-15.

Perhaps, but the test itself may not allow one to use different angles. The reflections from the interface between the wedge and test specimen will always be present to a certain degree during angle beam testing by the contact method. However, they should create no problems once it is realized that this is an ever-present phenomena.

Turn back to page 6-13.

A small surface wave component is transmitted in all directions from the transducer. When the transducer is close to an edge of the specimen, a reflection will be obtained that may be interpreted as a discontinuity. This type of nonrelevant indication can be easily identified, since movement of the transducer will cause the surface wave indication to move across the display with the movement of the transducer.

Is the following statement true or false? It will be possible to detect discontinuities even if the transducer is close enough to the edge of the test specimen so that spurious surface wave indications are received.

True . . . . **Page 6-12**

False . . . . **Page 6-16**

Your answer is not correct. It *will be possible* to detect discontinuities in the presence of unwanted surface wave indications. Once the spurious indication is identified as such, we can disregard it and look only for other indications. There will be many occasions when indications are present which are meaningless insofar as detection of discontinuities is concerned. The correct answer is "true."

Turn back to page 6-12.

You can determine if the reflection is from a surface wave by running a finger along the surface in front of the transducer. If the reflection is due to the presence of surface waves, the wave will be damped by your finger. To determine crack location, move the transducer until the discontinuity indication coincides with the indication from the initial pulse. At that point, the transducer wedge exit point is essentially over the crack.

Under which of the following conditions of angled sound beam transmission do you think you would be more likely to generate a surface wave component?

Small angle of incidence; i.e., 45° . . . . **Page 6-18**
Large angle of incidence; i.e., 70° . . . . **Page 6-21**

Your answer is not correct. At a small angle of incidence the sound beam will strike the surface of the test specimen closer to the perpendicular and there will be less refraction than if a larger angle is used. When there is least refraction, the surface wave component will be least. As the angle of incidence is increased, the surface wave component will increase until the second critical angle is reached when the refracted beam is composed entirely of surface waves in the test specimen.

Turn ahead to page 6-21.

Correct. Surface grinding *does not* need to be accomplished if sufficient sound energy is being transmitted into the specimen to obtain a back surface reflection. The surface wave reflection is identified as nonrelevant, so it can be disregarded and the specimen can be tested for valid discontinuities.

Turn to the next page.

Unwanted reflections can occur as a result of "mode conversion" in the test specimen. You learned that refraction and reflection can occur any time a sound beam strikes an interface between two mediums at an angle other than 90°. When this happens, as in the following illustration, the reflected beam inside the specimen will have both a longitudinal and shear component. The shear wave component can, at times, cause additional indications.

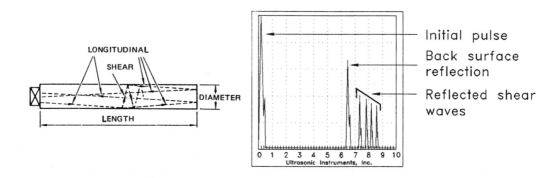

In the example illustrated above, a long bar is being tested. The reflected shear waves travel a longer distance than the longitudinal waves and, for this reason, will appear on the screen following the back surface reflection at regular intervals. They can be disregarded in evaluating discontinuity indications that occur between the front and back surface indications. Proper transducer selection will assist in reducing unwanted reflections such as those illustrated above.

At a given frequency, which of the following transducers will give less beam spread?

Small transducer . . . . **Page 6-23**
Large transducer . . . . **Page 6-24**

Right. A surface wave component is more likely to be generated during angle beam testing if you are using a *large* angle of incidence.

Unwanted surface wave components of the sound beam in the test specimen can also cause nonrelevant indications when the surface is rough. The surface of the test specimen may have been machined but, if surface grooves or machining marks exist, reflection will occur and result in apparent discontinuity indications.

These unwanted surface wave reflections again can be distinguished from valid discontinuity indications by running your finger along the test surface. If the indication is caused by surface waves, the waves will be damped by your finger and the indication amplitude diminished.

When testing a rough-machined specimen and a known nonrelevant indication due to the presence of surface waves is received, which of the following actions should be taken? Assume that a discernible back surface reflection is obtained.

Proceed with the test .... **Page 6-19**
Grind the surface .... **Page 6-22**

Your answer is not the best of the two possibilities. When a back surface reflection is received, you know enough sound energy is being transmitted into the specimen to locate a discontinuity if one is present.

The nonrelevant indication from the surface wave should be disregarded and the test continued. Under conditions where nonrelevant indications clutter the CRT to the extent that valid indications cannot be distinguished, you may have to smooth the surface. However, don't resort to grinding unless absolutely necessary.

Turn back to page 6-19.

Your selection is wrong. A small transducer produces more beam spread than a large one at a given frequency. In this case, selection of a large transducer will provide a narrower beam and the amount of internal mode conversion will be reduced.

Turn to the next page.

Correct. A large transducer will give you a narrower beam. With the narrower beam, unwanted internal mode conversion will be reduced.

Apparent discontinuity indications can be caused by reflection from surfaces in irregularly-shaped test specimens such as are illustrated below.

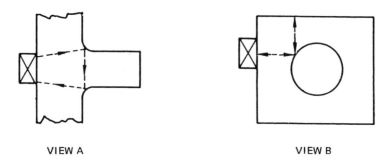

VIEW A   VIEW B

The possibility of reflections from fillets and corners must be taken into consideration when testing castings such as in View A above. Specimens with internal bore holes will also provide spurious indications as shown in View B.

When testing specimens such as those illustrated, the operator should examine the drawing of the article and select the point for making the test that will give the least amount of unwanted reflections.

Suppose a test of an irregularly-shaped specimen is being conducted. Which of the following actions should we take to confirm that an apparent discontinuity is actual or due to a reflection from a corner?

Test from a different part of the surface . . . . **Page 6-26**
Use shear wave techniques . . . . **Page 6-28**

This type of spurious indication can be identified easily, since the same type of indication will occur all along the length of the cylindrical specimen. Reflections from discontinuities, on the other hand, will cause a changing indication as the transducer is moved along the cylinder.

Which of the following methods will be *best* for lessening the spread of the sound beam transmitted into a cylindrical test specimen?

Use a smaller transducer . . . . **Page 6-27**
Use a curved, plexiglass shoe that fits the specimen contour . . . . **Page 6-29**

That's right. The operator should make a test from another location on the surface of the specimen in an effort to evaluate the indication as being either from an actual discontinuity or from a corner of the specimen.

Additional reflections following the back surface reflection can occur when tests are being made on cylindrical specimens, especially when the face of the transducer is not curved to fit the form of the specimen as illustrated.

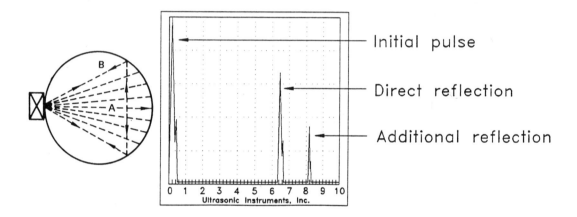

The beam spread of a sound wave depends on the size of the transmitting area of the transducer. When a flat transducer is placed on a curved surface, the transmitting area is very small and the beam spread will be practically 180°. Additional reflections will occur after the first back surface reflection. These reflections will occur sooner and more frequently with a smooth test surface. On a rough surface, such as a casting, the roughness of the surface will scatter the sound and the additional reflections may not be noticed.

Turn back to page 6-25.

A smaller transducer may not help to any great extent. As long as the surface of the transducer is flat, there will still be a large spreading of the sound beam. Remember, the smaller the transducer, the greater the beam spread and, in this case, the effective transmitting area of the transducer that touches the test specimen is smaller. You have gained nothing. The best thing to do is to use a plexiglass wedge that fits the contour of the cylindrical specimen.

Turn ahead to page 6-29.

Your answer is not correct. Use of shear wave techniques would *not* be an aid in confirming whether an indication is due to a discontinuity or due to the shape of the specimen. You should make the test from another location on the test surface and try to avoid reflections from a corner.

Turn back to page 6-26.

Correct. A smaller transducer won't do the job, since it will cause more spreading of the sound beam if anything. The only practical method of lessening the spread of the sound beam will be to use a plastic shoe that fits the contour of the cylindrical specimen.

Now we will consider the effects of internal grain structure on sound transmission and the types of indications that might be obtained with coarse grain structures.

There are times when sound transmission in a material is impossible, even with the strongest possible signal and the maximum gain of the test instrument. Under such conditions it may not be possible to receive a reflection from the back surface and system sensitivity for locating discontinuities is practically zero. It may be possible to improve the sound transmission capability of the system by using a lower frequency.

When a situation such as that described above occurs, what type of grain structure is indicated?

Fine . . . . **Page 6-30**
Coarse . . . . **Page 6-32**

You guessed, didn't you?   This particular point has been discussed previously. Coarse grain structure scatters and absorbs the sound beam. If the grain structure is coarse enough, the sound beam will be completely scattered and/or absorbed and there will be no reflection back to the transducer. On the other hand, fine grain structure offers little opposition to the passage of the sound beam and maximum transmission efficiency is obtained.

Turn ahead to page 6-32.

Very good. You remembered that wavelength is inversely proportional to frequency. So if the frequency is decreased, the wavelength is increased. This would provide for improved penetration at the expense of discontinuity detectability.

The last nonrelevant indication to be considered is one that will be received accidentally and is caused by the use of too much couplant. This type of indication will move slowly along the baseline or change amplitude as couplant flows along the surface of the test specimen. It is usually encountered when using angle beam techniques in contact testing.

What can we do to minimize this type of nonrelevant indication during testing?

Use the correct frequency .... **Page 6-33**
Do not use an excessive amount of couplant .... **Page 6-35**

Excellent. If the grain structure is sufficiently coarse, the sound beam will be scattered and/or absorbed and there will be no reflection back to the transducer for display on the test instrument.

If the test is attempted at a high frequency, coarse grain structures may also cause reflections that appear across the width of the display as illustrated.

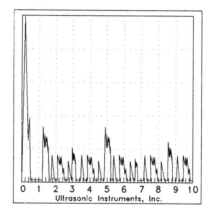

Due to their irregularity, it is not difficult to identify these indications; however, identification of discontinuity indications will be very difficult, if not impossible. The only thing that can be done to eliminate or reduce the effect of these unwanted reflections is to lower the frequency and change the direction of the sound beam.

The relationship of wavelength to size of the grain in a specimen is the factor that can cause or minimize reflections such as those illustrated above.

The size of the grain in a specimen will remain constant; therefore, as the frequency is lowered, wavelength:

increases . . . . **Page 6-31**
decreases . . . . **Page 6-34**

What happened? You shouldn't have turned to this page. You have an indication that slowly moves across the CRT or changes in amplitude. This is an indication that you are generating a reflection caused by excess couplant. Changing the frequency will be of no help. Removal of excess couplant will solve the problem.

Turn ahead to page 6-35.

Your answer is not correct. You have forgotten that "wavelength" is equal to the velocity of sound divided by the frequency, or that wavelength is *inversely proportional* to frequency. So, in this case, the frequency is being decreased and the wavelength will have to increase to satisfy the mathematical relationship of wavelength, velocity, and frequency.

Turn back to page 6-31.

That is correct.   The operator merely needs to exercise caution in the application of couplant and troubles with nonrelevant indications that move or change amplitude will be minimized.

All of the various types of nonrelevant indications that have been covered come from the test method itself with the exception of those covered in the beginning of the discussion that are a result of equipment troubles.

These indications will cause no difficulties in interpreting ultrasonic test results so long as it is understood that not all indications indicate a discontinuity in the test specimen. Also, you need to remember the basic principles of isolation for these apparent discontinuity indications to separate valid indications from invalid indications.

Turn to the next page for a short review.

CHAPTER REVIEW

_____ 1. The _____ control on a test instrument may be used to decrease the amplitude of low amplitude indications, including noise.

    A. range
    B. gain
    C. delay
    D. reject

_____ 2. An apparent discontinuity that broadens the baseline is caused by:

    A. attenuation.
    B. couplant.
    C. noise.
    D. surface waves.

_____ 3. "Wrap around" in the test specimen is caused when one sound pulse is not fully attenuated before a second pulse is transmitted. This spurious indication can be reduced by adjusting the _____ of the pulser.

    A. height
    B. repetition rate
    C. frequency
    D. pulse width

_____ 4. Unwanted reflections from the wedge of an angle beam transducer can be minimized by the _____ of the wedge.

A. width
B. angle
C. color
D. design (shape)

_____ 5. A loose or defective crystal in the transducer may produce a/an _____ effect on the CRT.

A. ringing
B. discoloration
C. inversion
D. attenuation

_____ 6. During straight beam or angle beam testing on rough surfaces, a small _____ wave component may be transmitted in all directions from the transducer. If this wave component strikes an edge of the specimen or a crack, a reflection will occur and provide a spurious discontinuity indication.

A. shear
B. plate
C. surface
D. longitudinal

_____ 7. Suppose you are testing a rough-machined surface with two transducers; one for receiving and one for transmitting. The transducers should be oriented _____ to the grooves.

A. parallel
B. perpendicular
C. diagonally
D. backwards

_____ 8. A curved, plexiglass wedge that fits the curvature of a cylindrical specimen will cause a _____ sound beam to be transmitted into the specimen.

A. wide
B. cylindrical
C. oblong
D. narrow

_____ 9. A _____ grain structure will scatter and/or absorb ultrasound to the extent that it may not be possible to conduct tests on some specimens.

A. fine
B. coarse
C. unique
D. dendritic

_____   10.   An indication that moves slowly with respect to the front surface indication and may change amplitude may be caused by the use of too much:

A.   couplant.
B.   gain.
C.   range.
D.   voltage.

Turn to the next page for answers to these review questions.

ANSWERS TO REVIEW QUESTIONS
FOR CHAPTER 6

Question & Answer		Reference Page(s)
1.	D	6-2
2.	C	6-2
3.	B	6-9
4.	D	6-8
5.	A	6-5
6.	C	6-13
7.	A	6-21
8.	D	6-29
9.	B	6-29
10.	A	6-31, 6-35

Turn to the next page.

Congratulations! You have just completed the third and final volume of the programmed instruction course on ultrasonic testing.

You may want to evaluate your knowledge of the material presented in this handbook; therefore, a set of self-test questions are included at the back of the book. The answers can be found at the end of the test.

Again, we want to emphasize that the test is for *your own* evaluation of *your* knowledge of the subject. If you elect to take the test, be honest with yourself - don't refer to the answers until you have finished. Then you will have a meaningful measure of your knowledge.

Since it is a self evaluation, there is no grade and no passing score. If you find that you have trouble in some part of the test, it is up to you to review the material until you are satisfied that you know it.

Turn to page A-1 and begin.

APPENDIX A

VOLUME III - APPLICATIONS

SELF-TEST

1. The test system which relies on reflected energy to find discontinuities is called:

   A. through-transmission.
   B. pulse-echo.
   C. longitudinal wave.
   D. continuous wave.

2. The test system that uses either pulsed or continuous sound and indicates discontinuities as a reduction in received energy is called:

   A. contact testing.
   B. longitudinal wave testing.
   C. pulse-echo testing.
   D. through-transmission testing.

3. The ultrasonic test where the transducer is coupled to the test specimen through a thin layer of couplant is called:

   A. immersion testing.
   B. contact testing.
   C. coupled-wave testing.
   D. through-transmission testing.

_____ 4. The test technique where both the transducer and the test specimen are placed in a tank filled with a liquid (water) is called:

A. contact testing.
B. through-transmission testing.
C. submerged testing.
D. immersion testing.

_____ 5. The ability of an ultrasonic system to detect discontinuities is *not* affected by the surface condition, shape, or metallurgical characteristics of a specimen to be tested.

A. True
B. False

_____ 6. Pulse-echo testing provides specific data on the relative size of the discontinuity and its sound-path distance.

A. True
B. False

_____ 7. The requirement that the transmitting and receiving transducers have to be precisely aligned on the test specimen is a disadvantage of:

A. contact testing.
B. longitudinal wave testing.
C. pulse-echo testing.
D. through-transmission testing.

8. Which of the following factors is an *advantage* of contact testing over immersion testing?

    A. Bulky test apparatus
    B. Higher frequencies may be used
    C. Better resolution
    D. Greater beam penetration

9. Which of the following factors is a *disadvantage* of contact testing?

    A. Decreased beam penetration power
    B. Portability
    C. Difficulty in maintaining a uniform acoustical coupling
    D. Confined to high-frequency testing only

10. Which of the following factors is an *advantage* of immersion testing over the contact technique?

    A. Greater beam penetration power
    B. Portability
    C. Lower test frequencies may be used
    D. Angulation for unfavorably oriented discontinuities

11. Which of the following is a *disadvantage* of immersion testing?

    A. Reduced transducer wear
    B. Better resolution
    C. Portability
    D. Angulation ability

12. Equipment selection and operation are parameters of the ultrasonic test system that are controlled by the operator.

 A. True
 B. False

13. To improve the ultrasonic test of a given specimen, which of the following may be modified?

 A. Specimen shape
 B. Adjustment of instrument controls
 C. Specimen material
 D. Specimen heat treat

14. The requirements of an ultrasonic test are:

 A. determined by operator judgment.
 B. established by the reference standard block used.
 C. outlined in the test procedure.
 D. None of the above.

15. Calibration of ultrasonic test instruments is based on reflections received from reference standards containing simulated discontinuities of known size.

 A. True
 B. False

16. Any precisely-machined reference standard block may be used in calibrating a test instrument for testing a given test specimen.

    A. True
    B. False

17. In ultrasonics, pulse-echo testing is more widely used than through-transmission testing.

    A. True
    B. False

18. A particular advantage of through-transmission testing is that:

    A. no couplant is required.
    B. the depth of a discontinuity can be easily determined.
    C. only one transducer is required.
    D. None of the above.

19. Proper test equipment selection is dependent upon the:

    A. test specimen geometry.
    B. metallurgical structure of the specimen.
    C. overall test situation.
    D. surface condition of the test specimen.

20. Which of the following frequencies would probably result in the greatest attenuation loss?

    A.   1 MHz
    B.   10 MHz
    C.   15 MHz
    D.   25 MHz

21. The characteristics of the internal grain structure of a test specimen need to be considered when selecting the test frequency.

    A.   True
    B.   False

22. To test large, flat specimens, the transducer should have:

    A.   an acoustical lens.
    B.   a small surface area.
    C.   a large surface area.
    D.   a curved surface.

23. In order to find the smallest discontinuities during a test:

    A.   use the lowest frequency possible.
    B.   use the highest frequency possible.
    C.   use through-transmission testing.
    D.   use a small transducer.

24. Transducers incorporating a plastic wedge are commonly used in straight beam testing.

   A. True
   B. False

25. The acoustical impedance of an ideal couplant should be between that of the transducer and the test specimen.

   A True
   B. False

26. The choice of a couplant is largely dependent upon the surface condition of the test specimen.

   A. True
   B. False

27. Loss of back surface reflection is evidence that sound is not being returned to the:

   A. discontinuity.
   B. transducer.
   C. test specimen.
   D. back surface.

28. A short pulse length results in:

   A. less instrument sensitivity.
   B. less penetration power.
   C. better near surface sensitivity.
   D. increased penetration power.

29. In contact testing, shear waves may be produced in a test specimen by:

   A. placing an X-cut quartz crystal on the specimen and coupling with oil.
   B. using two transducers, one on each side of the specimen.
   C. using a shear-cut lens on the transducer.
   D. using an angle beam transducer.

30. The first critical incident angle for longitudinal waves is the point at which:

   A. the reflected angle is zero degrees.
   B. the refracted angle of the longitudinal wave mode is parallel to the surface.
   C. the longitudinal wave mode is totally reflected.
   D. both longitudinal and shear waves are transmitted into the specimen.

31. What wave is developed when the shear wave mode is refracted 90°?

A. Longitudinal wave
B. Surface wave
C. Transverse wave
D. Transitional wave

32. Ultrasonic waves which travel around a gradual curve with little or no reflection from the curve are called:

A. longitudinal waves.
B. shear waves.
C. surface waves.
D. transverse waves.

33. Plate waves are used to test:

A. castings.
B. forgings.
C. bar stock.
D. thin sheet.

34. With reference to single-transducer pulse-echo testing, two-transducer pulse-echo testing has better:

A. near surface resolution.
B. specimen penetration power.
C. resolution at all depths.
D. sensitivity at all depths.

35. Ultrasonic testing of castings is often not possible because of:

A. rough surfaces.
B. small grain structure.
C. coarse grain structure.
D. irregular shape.

36. Which of the following materials is most likely to produce the greatest amount of sound attenuation over a given distance?

A. Hand forging
B. Coarse-grained casting
C. Extrusion
D. Fine-grained material

37. It is normal practice in testing bar stock to use both axial and radial tests (test through both the length and the width of the specimen).

A. True
B. False

38. In straight beam contact testing, with the sound beam entering a flat specimen (such as a plate from one of the surfaces), which of the following type of discontinuity will probably be detected?

   A. Radial-type discontinuity with major dimension along the length but radially oriented to the surface
   B. Transverse-type discontinuity at an angle to the surface
   C. Laminations with major dimensions parallel to the surface
   D. Porosity

39. A *gross* check of plate or sheet consists of marking off a grid pattern on the material, either real or imaginary, and then testing each grid square using:

   A. a transducer wheel.
   B. a focused transducer.
   C. an angle beam transducer.
   D. a straight beam transducer.

40. Before using an angle beam transducer for testing plate, a reference notch must be evaluated to determine the size of any discontinuities that might be found.

   A. True
   B. False

41. The most common application of ultrasonic tests using shear waves is:

A. testing large, round specimens.
B. determining elastic properties of materials.
C. detection of laminations in rolled plate.
D. detection of discontinuities in pipe, tubing, and welds.

42. A notch-type reference standard for testing of tubing should be machined on:

A. the outer surface only.
B. the inner surface only.
C. both inner and outer surfaces.
D. All of the above.

43. During weld testing, the fusion zone may return a reflection that is similar to reflections from discontinuities.

A. True
B. False

44. The term "skip distance" refers to the bouncing of a sound beam between opposite material boundaries in angle beam testing. This distance will change as material thickness changes.

A. True
B. False

45. Skip distance is determined by:

A. the angle of reflection.
B. the test frequency used.
C. the pulse width used.
D. the angle of refraction.

46. Generally, the best ultrasonic testing technique for detecting discontinuities oriented along the fusion zone in a welded plate is the:

A. contact technique using surface waves.
B. straight beam technique using longitudinal waves.
C. angle beam technique using shear waves.
D. straight beam technique using plate waves.

47. When using the formula a = W (sin α) to determine a discontinuity's physical location, the refracted angle must be first determined before any calculations can be made as to a discontinuity location.

A. True
B. False

48. The stainless steel IIW (International Institute of Welding) reference blocks can be used to test welds in any material.

A. True
B. False

49. Direct-reading ultrasonic calculators are used to locate discontinuities in plate when:

A. transducer incident beam angle and plate sound velocity are known.
B. plate thickness and transducer wedge velocity are known.
C. transducer wedge and plate velocities are known.
D. plate thickness and transducer refraction angle are known.

50. A wetting agent is used in immersion test tanks to prevent the formation of small air bubbles that could produce confusing reflections.

A. True
B. False

51. The carriage used in immersion testing supports the:

A. immersion tank.
B. equipment operator.
C. scanner tube and manipulator.
D. test instrument.

52. The tubular device held by the manipulator is called a:

A. vertical probe.
B. wand.
C. scanner tube.
D. transducer.

53. Which of the following is an advantage of a focused transducer over a conventional transducer used in immersion testing?

    A.   Less sensitivity to small discontinuities
    B.   Increased resolving power
    C.   Increased effects from surface roughness
    D.   Greater penetrating power

54. If a test specimen is too large to be placed in an immersion tank, the advantages of immersion testing can still be attained by using a "bubbler" (water column).

    A.   True
    B.   False

55. In immersion testing, the water multiples that may be seen on the CRT between the front and back surface reflections can be eliminated by:

    A.   using a different frequency transducer.
    B.   increasing the distance from the transducer to the test specimen.
    C.   using a contour correction lens.
    D.   decreasing instrument sensitivity.

56. A general rule of thumb in determining the correct water distance to use in immersion testing is that the water distance should be:

A. equal to the thickness of the test specimen.
B. 1/2 the thickness of the test specimen.
C. 1/4 the thickness of the test specimen plus 1/4 inch (6.3 mm).
D. equal to the thickness of the test specimen plus 1/4 inch (6.3 mm).

57. In immersion testing, the transducer will be transmitting its sound beam perpendicular to the test surface when _____ is received on the CRT.

A. minimum back surface amplitude
B. elimination of water multiples
C. maximum front surface reflection
D. maximum initial pulse amplitude

58. In immersion testing, the water distance between the transducer and the test specimen should be:

A. as small as possible.
B. as great as possible.
C. the same as that used for standardization.
D. twice the specimen thickness.

59. In immersion testing, the area at which a sound beam enters a specimen can be determined by using a straight-edged "metal spoon."

A. True
B. False

60. During immersion testing it is often necessary to angulate the transducer when a discontinuity is located to:

A. avoid a large number of back reflections that could interfere with a normal test pattern.
B. obtain a maximum response if the discontinuity is not originally oriented perpendicular to the sound beam.
C. obtain the maximum number of front surface reflections.
D. obtain a discontinuity indication that is the same height as the indication from the flat-bottomed hole in a reference block.

61. Either longitudinal or shear waves can be used in immersion testing of cylindrically-shaped specimens.

A. True
B. False

62. Thin-walled tubing is most effectively tested using:

A. longitudinal waves.
B. shear waves.
C. articulated waves.
D. compressional waves.

63. In immersion testing using the angle beam technique, the specimen front surface indication will be:

A. high in amplitude.
B. small but well-defined.
C. strong and well-defined.
D. small and poorly-defined.

64. A nonrelevant indication that appears like a discontinuity indication but is not synchronized with the baseline and moves from left to right will be due to:

A. material structure interference.
B. loose transducer crystal.
C. electrical interference.
D. interference from refraction.

65. A loose or defective transducer crystal will produce a ringing effect.

A. True
B. False

66. In contact testing, spurious indications resulting from transducer wedge interference can be isolated simply by lifting the transducer off the test specimen and seeing if the indication remains.

A. True
B. False

67. In straight beam testing using two transducers, a discontinuity indication that can be damped out by placing a finger on the surface is the result of:

A. longitudinal waves striking a discontinuity.
B. specimen grain structure.
C. surface waves traveling on the test specimen surface.
D. electrical interference.

68. An ultrasonic operator should primarily look for indications appearing to the left of the back surface reflection because:

A. they are the strongest and most easily seen.
B. they determine material thickness.
C. they determine what test specification may be used.
D. they are most likely to be caused by discontinuities.

69. In testing long specimens, spurious signals may result if the sound beam spreads into the sides of the material before reaching the back surface.

   A.   True
   B.   False

70. Interference from fine grain in a test specimen can sometimes be distinguished by numerous reflections following the front surface indication.

   A.   True
   B.   False

71. In contact angle beam testing, an indication that moves slowly across the CRT or changes amplitude can be the result of:

   A.   not enough couplant.
   B.   too much couplant.

72. Which of the following wave modes is used for the tip diffraction technique?

   A.   Plate
   B.   Longitudinal
   C.   Surface
   D.   Shear and longitudinal

73. When applying tip diffraction techniques to determine the through-wall dimension of a crack in plate, the tip signal will _____ in relation to the corner trap signal as the crack height increases.

A. remain at the same CRT location
B. move right
C. move left
D. appear behind and increase in amplitude

74. In the following illustration, which view indicates a 0.3 inch (7.6 mm) through-wall crack? Assume a display calibrated to 0.1 inch (2.5 mm) per division.

A. View A
B. View B

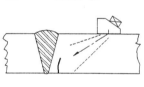 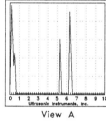 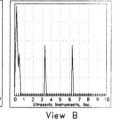

View A   View B

75. In the following illustration the back wall indication is at 6.5 inches (165.1 mm). What is the sound-path distance to the discontinuity?

A. 0.4 inches (10.2 mm)
B. 3.4 inches (86.4 mm)
C. 4.1 inches (104.1 mm)

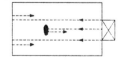 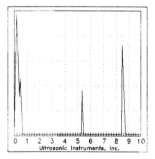

Turn to the next page for answers to these questions.

ANSWERS TO VOLUME III SELF-TEST

Question & Answer		Reference Page(s)	Question & Answer		Reference Page(s)
1.	B	1-2	21.	A	2-14
2.	D	1-5	22.	C	2-16
3.	B	1-10	23.	B	2-13
4.	D	1-10	24.	B	2-24
5.	B	1-14	25.	A	2-26
6.	A	1-22	26.	A	2-23, 2-26
7.	D	1-15	27.	B	2-31, 2-32
8.	D	1-21	28.	B	2-32
9.	C	1-25	29.	D	2-33, 2-36
10.	D	1-24	30.	B	2-38
11.	C	1-27	31.	B	2-49
12.	A	1-34	32.	C	2-51
13.	B	1-34	33.	D	2-53
14.	C	1-36	34.	A	2-59, 2-61
15.	A	1-40	35.	C	3-1
16.	B	1-42	36.	B	3-1
17.	A	2-2	37.	A	3-7
18.	D	2-6	38.	C	3-13
19.	C	2-9	39.	D	3-20
20.	D	2-14	40.	A	3-19

Turn to the next page.

ANSWERS TO THE VOLUME III SELF-TEST

Answers		Reference Page(s)	Answers		Reference Page(s)
41.	D	3-29	61.	A	5-7
42.	C	3-40	62.	B	5-19
43.	A	3-41	63.	D	5-30
44.	A	3-47	64.	C	6-4
45.	D	3-47	65.	A	6-5
46.	C	3-41	66.	A	6-11
47.	A	3-47	67.	C	6-21
48.	B	3-70	68.	D	6-20
49.	D	3-74	69.	A	6-20
50.	A	4-2	70.	B	6-32
51.	C	4-4	71.	B	6-31
52.	C	4-4	72.	D	3-87
53.	B	4-15	73.	C	3-89
54.	A	4-24	74.	B	3-90, 3-92
55.	B	4-27	75.	C	1-1, 1-4
56.	C	4-31			
57.	C	4-38			
58.	C	4-40			
59.	A	4-42, 4-43			
60.	B	4-41			

Review and re-test as you feel the need.

APPENDIX B

GLOSSARY

A-scan Display   A display in which the received signal is displayed as a vertical displacement from the horizontal sweep time trace, while the horizontal distance between any two signals represents the sound path distance (or time of travel) between the two.

Absorption Coefficient, Linear   The fractional decrease in transmitted intensity per unit of absorber thickness. It is usually designated by the symbol μ and expressed in units of cm^{-1}.

Acceptance Standard   A control specimen containing natural or artificial discontinuities that are well defined and, in size or extent, similar to the maximum acceptable in the product. Also may refer to the document defining acceptable discontinuity size limits.

Acoustic Impedance   The factor which controls the propagation of an ultrasonic wave at a boundary interface. It is the product of the material density and the acoustic wave velocity within that material.

Amplifier   A device to increase or amplify electrical impulses.

Amplitude, Indication   The vertical height of a received indication, measured from base-to-peak or peak-to-peak.

Angle Beam Testing   A testing method in which transmission is at an angle to the sound entry surface.

Angle of Incidence   The angle between the incident (transmitted) beam and a normal to the boundary interface.

Angle of Reflection   The angle between the reflected beam and a normal to the boundary interface.   The angle of reflection is equal to the angle of incidence.

Angle of Refraction   The angle between the refracted rays of an ultrasonic beam and the normal (or perpendicular line) to the refracting surface.

Angle Transducer   A transducer that transmits or receives the acoustic energy at an acute angle to the surface to achieve a specific effect such as the setting up of shear or surface waves in the part being inspected.

Anisotropic   A condition in which properties of a medium (velocity, for example) vary according to the direction in which they are measured.

Array Transducer   A transducer made up of several piezoelectric elements individually connected so that the signals they transmit or receive may be treated separately or combined as desired.

ANSI   American National Standards Institute

API   American Petroleum Institute

ASME   American Society of Mechanical Engineers

ASNT   American Society for Nondestructive Testing

ASTM   American Society for Testing and Materials

Attenuation Coefficient   A factor which is determined by the degree of scatter or absorption of ultrasound energy per unit distance traveled.

Attenuation   The loss in acoustic energy which occurs between any two points of travel. This loss may be due to absorption, reflection, scattering, etc.

Attenuator   A device for measuring attenuation, usually calibrated in decibels (dB).

B-scan Display   A data presentation method that represents a cross-sectional or end view display of the test article.

Back Reflection   The signal received from the back surface of a test object. Also referred to as back wall reflection.

Back Scatter   Scattered signals that are directed back to the transmitter/receiver.

Background Noise   Extraneous signals caused by signal sources within the ultrasonic testing system, including the material in test.

Baseline   The horizontal line across the bottom of the CRT created by the sweep circuit.

Basic Calibration   The procedure of standardizing an instrument using calibration reflectors described in an application document.

Beam Exit/Index Point   The point on a transducer (primarily angle beam) indicating the physical location through which the emergent beam axis passes.

Beam Spread   The divergence of the sound beam as it travels through a medium.

Bi-modal The propagation of sound in a test article where at least a shear wave and a longitudinal wave exists. The operation of angle beam testing at less than first critical angle.

Boundary Indication A reflection of an ultrasonic beam from an interface.

Broad Banded Having a relatively wide frequency bandwidth. Used to describe pulses which display a wide frequency spectrum and receivers capable of amplifying them.

C-scan A data presentation method yielding a plan (top) view through the scanned surface of the part. Through gating, only indications arising from the interior of the test object are indicated.

Calibration To determine or mark the graduations of the ultrasonic system's display relative to a known standard or reference.

Calibration Reflector A reflector with a known dimensioned surface established to provide an accurately reproducible reference.

Collimator An attachment designed to reduce the ultrasonic beam spread.

Compensator An electrical matching network to compensate for circuit impedance differences.

Compressional Wave A wave in which the particle motion or vibration is in the same direction as the propagated wave (longitudinal wave).

Contact Testing A technique of testing in which the transducer contacts the test surface, either directly or through a thin layer of couplant.

Contact Transducer A transducer which is coupled to a test surface either directly or through a thin film of couplant.

Continuous Wave A wave that continues without interruption.

Contracted Sweep A contraction of the horizontal sweep on the viewing screen of the ultrasonic instrument. Contraction of this sweep permits viewing reflections occurring over a greater sound-path distance or duration of time.

Corner Effect The strong reflection obtained when an ultrasonic beam is directed toward the inner section of two or three mutually perpendicular surfaces.

Couplant A substance used between the face of the transducer and test surface to permit or improve transmission of ultrasonic energy across this boundary or interface. Primarily used to remove the air in the interface.

Critical Angle The incident angle of the sound beam beyond which a specific refracted mode of vibration no longer exists.

Cross Talk An unwanted condition in which acoustic energy is coupled from the transmitting crystal to the receiving crystal without propagating along the intended path through the material.

Damping (transducer) Limiting the duration of vibration in the search unit by either electrical or mechanical means.

Dead Zone The distance in a material from the sound entry surface to the nearest inspectable sound path.

Decibel (dB) The logarithmic expression of a ratio of two amplitudes or intensities of acoustic energy.

Defect/Flaw   A material discontinuity whose size, shape, orientation or location make it detrimental to the useful service of the test object or component.

Defect Indication   The oscilloscope presentation of the energy returned by a rejectable flaw in the material.

Delamination   A laminar discontinuity, generally an area of unbonded materials.

Delay Line   A material (liquid or solid) placed in front of a transducer to cause a time delay between the initial pulse and the front surface reflection.

Delayed Sweep   A means of delaying the start of horizontal sweep, thereby eliminating the presentation of early response data.

Delta Effect   Acoustic energy re-radiated by a discontinuity.

Detectability The ability of the ultrasonic system to locate a discontinuity.

Diffraction   The deflection, or "bending," of a wave front when passing the edge or edges of a discontinuity.

Diffuse Reflection   Scattered, incoherent reflections caused by rough surfaces or associate interface reflection of ultrasonic waves from irregularities of the same order of magnitude or greater than the wavelength.

Discontinuity   An interruption or change in the physical structure or characteristics of a material.

Dispersion, Sound Scattering of an ultrasonic beam as a result of diffuse reflection from a highly-irregular surface.

Distance Amplitude Correction (DAC)   Compensation of gain as a function of time for difference in amplitude of reflections from equal reflectors at different sound travel distances.   Also referred to as time corrected gain (TCG), time variable gain (TVG) and sensitivity time control (STC).

Divergence   Spreading of ultrasonic waves after leaving search unit, and is a function of diameter and frequency.

Dual-Element Technique   The technique of ultrasonic testing using two transducers with one acting as the transmitter and one as the receiver.

Dual-Element Transducer   A single transducer housing containing two piezoelectric elements, one for transmitting and one for receiving.

Echo   See **Boundary Indication**.

Effective Penetration   The maximum depth in a material at which the ultrasonic transmission is sufficient for proper detection of discontinuities.

Electrical Noise   Extraneous signals caused by externally radiated electrical signals or from electrical interferences within the ultrasonic instrumentation.

Electromagnetic Acoustic Transducer (EMAT)   A device using the magneto effect to generate and receive acoustic signals for ultrasonic nondestructive tests.

Evaluation   The process of deciding the severity of a condition after an indication has been interpreted.   Evaluation determines if the test object should be rejected, repaired, accepted, or replaced.

Far Field The region beyond the near field in which areas of high and low acoustic intensity cease to occur.

First Leg The sound path beginning at the exit point of the probe and extending to the point of contact opposite the examination surface when performing angle beam testing.

Focused Transducer A transducer with a concave face which converges the acoustic beam to a focal point or line at a defined distance from the face.

Focusing Concentration or convergence of energy into a smaller beam.

Fraunhofer Zone See **Far Field**.

Frequency Number of complete cycles of a wave motion passing a given point in a unit time (1 second); number of times a vibration is repeated at the same point in the same direction per unit time (usually per second).

Fresnel Field See **Near Field**.

Gate An electronic means to monitor an associated segment of time, distance, or impulse.

Ghost An indication which has no direct relation to reflected pulses from discontinuities in the materials being tested.

Hertz (Hz) One cycle per second.

Horizontal Sweep See **Baseline**.

Horizontal Linearity   A measure of the proportionality between the positions of the indications appearing on the baseline and the positions of their sources.

Immersion Testing A technique of testing, using a liquid as an ultrasonic couplant, in which the test part and at least the transducer face is immersed in the couplant and the transducer is not in contact with the test part.

Impedance (acoustic)   A material characteristic defined as a product of particle velocity and material density.

Indication (ultrasonics)   The signal displayed or read on the ultrasonic systems display.

Initial Pulse   The first indication which may appear on the screen. This indication represents the emission of ultrasonic energy from the crystal face (main bang).

Interface   The physical boundary between two adjacent acoustic mediums.

Insonification   Irradiation with sound.

Interpretation   The determination of the source and relevancy of an indication.

Isotropy A condition in which significant medium properties (velocity, for example) are the same in all directions.

Lamb Wave   A type of ultrasonic vibration guided by parallel surfaces of thin mediums capable of propagation in different modes.

Linearity (area)   A system response in which a linear relationship exists between amplitude of response and the discontinuity sizes being evaluated (necessarily limited by the size of the ultrasonic beam).

Linearity (depth)   A system response where a linear relationship exists with varying depth for a constant size discontinuity.

Longitudinal Wave   See **Compressional Wave**.

Longitudinal Wave Velocity   The unit speed of propagation of a longitudinal (compressional) wave through a material.

Loss of Back Reflection   Absence of or a significant reduction of an indication from the back surface of the article being inspected.

Major Screen Divisions The vertical graticule used to divide the CRT into 10 equal horizontal segments.

Manipulator   A device used to orient the transducer assembly. As applied to immersion techniques, it provides either angular or normal incidence and fixes the transducer-to-part distance.

Material Noise Extraneous signals caused by the structure of the material being tested.

Miniature Angle Beam Block A specific type of reference standard used primarily for the angle beam method, but also used for straight beam and surface wave tests.

Minor Screen Divisions The vertical graticule used to divide the CRT into 50 equal segments. Each major screen division is divided into 5 equal segments or minor divisions.

Mode Conversion   The change of ultrasonic wave propagation upon reflection or refraction at acute angles at an interface.

Mode   The manner in which acoustic energy is propagated through a material as characterized by the particle motion of the wave.

Multiple Back Reflections   Repetitive indications from the back surface of the material being examined.

Nanosecond   One billionth (10^{-9}) of a second.

Narrow Banded   A relative term denoting a restricted range of frequency response.

Near Field   A distance immediately in front of a transducer composed of complex and changing wave front characteristics.   Also known as the Fresnel field.

Node   The point on the examination surface where the V-path begins or ends. (See **V-path**)

Noise   Any undesired indications that tend to interfere with the interpretation or processing of the ultrasonic information; also referred to as "grass."

Nonrelevant Indication   See **Ghost**.

Normal Incidence   A condition where the angle of incidence is zero.

Orientation   The angular relationship of a surface, plane, defect axis, etc., to a reference plane or sound entry surface.

Penetration (ultrasonic)   Propagation of ultrasonic energy through an article. See **Effective Penetration**.

Phased Array   A mosaic of probe elements in which the timing of the element's excitation can be individually controlled to produce certain desired effects, such as steering the beam axis or focusing the beam.

Piezoelectric Effect   The characteristic of certain materials to generate electrical charges when subjected to mechanical vibrations and, conversely, to generate mechanical vibrations when subjected to electrical pulses.

Pitch-Catch   See **Two-Probe Method**.

Polarized Ceramics   Ceramic materials that are sintered (pressed), heated (approximately 1000°C), and polarized by applying a direct voltage of a few thousand volts per centimeter of thickness. The polarization is the process that makes these ceramics piezoelectric.   Includes sodium bismuth titanate, lead metaniobate, and several materials based on lead zirconate titanate (PZT).

Presentation   The method used to show ultrasonic information. This may include (among others) A-, B-, or C-scans displayed on various types of recorders, CRTs, LCDs or computerized displays.

Probe   Transducer or search unit.

Propagation   Advancement of a wave through a medium.

Pulse Echo Technique   An ultrasonic test technique using equipment which transmits a series of pulses separated by a constant period of time; i.e., energy is not sent out continuously.

Pulse Length   Time duration of the pulse from the search unit.

Pulse Rate   For the pulse echo technique, the number of pulses transmitted in a unit of time (also called pulse repetition rate).

Radio Frequency Display (RF)   The presentation of unrectified signals in a display.

Range   The maximum ultrasonic path length that is displayed.

Rarefaction   The thinning out or moving apart of the consistent particles in the propagating medium due to the relaxation phase of an ultrasonic cycle.   Opposite in its effect to compression.   The sound wave is composed of alternate compressions and refractions of the particles in a material.

Rayleigh Wave/Surface Wave   A wave that travels on or close to the surface and readily follows the curvature of the part being examined. Reflections occur only at sharp changes of direction of the surface.

Receiver   The section of the ultrasonic instrument that amplifies the electronic signals returning from the test specimen.   Also, the probe that receives the reflected signals.

Reference Blocks   A block or series of blocks of material containing artificial or actual discontinuities of one or more reflecting areas at one or more distances from the sound entry surface.   These are used for calibrating instruments and in defining the size and distance of discontinuous areas in materials.

Reflection   The characteristic of a surface to change the direction of propagating acoustic energy; the return of sound waves from surfaces.

Refraction A change in the direction and velocity of acoustic energy after it has passed at an acute angle through an interface between two different mediums.

Refractive Index The ratio of the velocity of a incident wave to the velocity of the refracted wave. It is a measure of the amount a wave will be refracted when it enters the second medium after leaving the first.

Reject/Suppression An instrument function or control used for reducing low amplitude signals. Use of this control may affect vertical linearity.

Relevant Indication In NDT, an indication from a discontinuity requiring evaluation.

Repetition Rate The rate at which the individual pulses of acoustic energy are generated; also **Pulse Rate**.

Resolving Power The capability measurement of an ultrasonic system to separate in time two closely spaced discontinuities or to separate closely spaced multiple reflections.

Resonance Technique A technique using the resonance principle for determining velocity, thickness or presence of laminar discontinuities.

Resonance The condition in which the frequency of a forcing vibration (ultrasonic wave) is the same as the natural vibration frequency of the propagation body (test object), resulting in large amplitude vibrations.

Saturation (scope) A term used to describe an indication of such a size as to exceed full screen height (100%).

Scanning (manual and automatic) The moving of the search unit or units along a test surface to obtain complete testing of a material.

Scattering   Dispersion of ultrasonic waves in a medium due to causes other than absorption. See **Diffuse** and **Dispersion**.

Second Leg   The sound path beginning at the point of contact on the opposite surface and extending to the point of contact on the examination surface when performing angle beam testing.

Sensitivity   The ability to detect small discontinuities at given distances. The level of amplification at which the receiving circuit in an ultrasonic instrument is set.

Shear Wave   The wave in which the particles of the medium vibrate in a direction perpendicular to the direction of propagation.

Signal-to-Noise Ratio (SNR)   The ratio of amplitudes of indications from the smallest discontinuity considered significant and those caused by random factors, such as heterogeneity in grain size, etc.

Skip Distance   In angle beam tests of plate, pipe, or welds, the linear or surface distance from the sound entry point to the first reflection point on the same surface.

Snell's Law   The law that defines the relationship between the angle of incidence and the angle of refraction across an interface, based on a change in ultrasonic velocity.

Specific Acoustic Impedance   A characteristic which acts to determine the amount of reflection which occurs at an interface and represents the wave velocity and the product of the density of the medium in which the wave is propagating.

Standardize   See **Calibration**.

Straight Beam   An ultrasonic wave traveling normal to the test surface.

Surface Wave   See **Rayleigh Wave**.

Sweep   The uniform and repeated movement of a spot across the screen of a CRT to form the baseline.

Through-Transmission   A test technique using two transducers in which the ultrasonic vibrations are emitted by one and received by the other, usually on the opposite side of the part.   The ratio of the magnitudes of vibrations transmitted and received is used as the criterion of soundness.

Tip Diffraction   The process by which a signal is generated from the tip (i.e., top of a fatigue crack) of a discontinuity through the interruption of an incident sound beam propagating through a material.

Transducer (search unit)   An assembly consisting basically of a housing, piezoelectric element, backing material, wear plate (optional) and electrical leads for converting electrical impulses into mechanical energy and vice versa.

Transmission Angle   The incident angle of the transmitted ultrasonic beam. It is zero degrees when the ultrasonic beam is perpendicular to the test surface.

Transmitter   The electrical circuit of an ultrasonic instrument that generates the pulses emitted to the search unit. Also the probe that emits ultrasonic signals.

Transverse Wave   See **Shear Wave**.

Two Probe Method   Use of two transducers for sending and receiving. May be either send-receive or through-transmission.

Ultrasonic Absorption A damping of ultrasonic vibrations that occurs when the wave transverses a medium.

Ultrasonic Spectrum The frequency span of elastic waves greater than the highest audible frequency, generally regarded as being higher than 20,000 hertz, to approximately 1000 megahertz.

Ultrasonic System The totality of components utilized to perform an ultrasonic test on a test article.

Ultrasonic Testing A nondestructive method of inspecting materials by the use of high-frequency sound waves into or through them.

V-path The path of the ultrasonic beam in the test object from the point of entry on the examination surface to the back surface and reflecting to the front surface again.

Velocity The speed at which sound travels through a medium.

Video Presentation A CRT presentation in which radio frequency signals have been rectified and usually filtered.

Water Path The distance from the face of the search unit to the entry surface of the material under test in immersion testing.

Wavelength The distance in the direction of propagation for a wave to go through one complete cycle.

Wedge/Shoe A device used to adapt a straight beam probe for use in a specific type of testing, including angle beam or surface wave tests and tests on curved surfaces.

Wrap Around Nonrelevant indications that appear on the CRT as a result of a short pulse repetition rate in the pulser circuit of the test instrument.

APPENDIX C

THREE-PLACE VALUES OF TRIGONOMETRIC FUNCTIONS							
Deg.	Sin	Tan	Sec	Csc	Cot	Cos	Deg.
0°	.000	.000	1.000	---	---	1.000	90°
1°	.017	.017	1.000	57.30	57.29	1.000	89°
2°	.035	.035	1.001	28.65	28.64	0.999	88°
3°	.052	.052	1.001	19.11	19.08	.999	87°
4°	.070	.070	1.002	14.34	14.30	.998	86°
5°	.087	.087	1.004	11.47	11.43	996	85°
6°	.105	.105	1.006	9.567	9.514	.995	84°
7°	.122	.123	1.008	8.206	8.144	.993	83°
8°	.139	.141	1.010	7.185	7.115	.990	82°
9°	.156	.158	1.012	6.392	6.314	.988	81°
10°	.174	.176	1.015	5.759	5.671	.985	80°
11°	.191	.194	1.019	5.241	5.145	.982	79°
12°	.208	.213	1.022	4.810	4.705	.978	78°
13°	.225	.231	1.026	4.445	4.331	.974	77°
14°	.242	.249	1.031	4.134	4.011	.970	76°
15°	.259	.268	1.035	3.864	3.732	.966	75°
16°	.276	.287	1.040	3.628	3.487	.961	74°
17°	.292	.306	1.046	3.420	3.271	.956	73°
18°	.309	.325	1.051	3.236	3.078	.951	72°
19°	.326	.344	1.058	3.072	2.904	.946	71°
20°	.342	.364	1.064	2.924	2.747	.940	70°
21°	.358	.384	1.071	2.790	2.605	.934	69°
22°	.375	.404	1.079	2.669	2.475	.927	68°
23°	.391	.424	1.086	2.559	2.356	.921	67°
24°	.407	.445	1.095	2.459	2.246	.914	66°
25°	.423	.466	1.103	2.366	2.145	.906	65°
26°	.438	.488	1.113	2.281	2.050	.899	64°
27°	.454	.510	1.122	2.203	1.963	.891	63°
28°	.469	.532	1.133	2.130	1.881	.883	62°
29°	.485	.554	1.143	2.063	1.804	.875	61°
30°	.500	.577	1.155	2.000	1.732	.866	60°
31°	.515	.601	1.167	1.942	1.664	.857	59°
32°	.530	.625	1.179	1.887	1.600	.848	58°
33°	.545	.649	1.192	1.836	1.540	.839	57°
34°	.559	.675	1.206	1.788	1.483	.829	56°
35°	.574	.700	1.221	1.743	1.428	.819	55°
36°	.588	.727	1.236	1.701	1.376	.809	54°
37°	.602	.754	1.252	1.662	1.327	.799	53°
38°	.616	.781	1.269	1.624	1.280	.788	52°
39°	.629	.810	1.287	1.589	1.235	.777	51°
40°	.643	.839	1.305	1.556	1.192	.766	50°
41°	.656	.869	1.325	1.524	1.150	.755	49°
42°	.669	.900	1.346	1.494	1.111	.743	48°
43°	.682	.933	1.367	1.466	1.072	.731	47°
44°	.695	0.966	1.390	1.440	1.036	.719	46°
45°	.707	1.000	1.414	1.414	1.000	.707	45°
Deg.	Cos	Cot	Csc	Sec	Tan	Sin	Deg.

APPENDIX D

Acoustic Properties of Materials

MATERIAL	DENSITY ρ = gm/cm³	LONGITUDINAL WAVES VELOCITY V_L = cm/μs	LONGITUDINAL WAVES IMPEDANCE Z_L = gm × 10³/cm²-s	SHEAR (TRANSVERSE) WAVES VELOCITY V_T = cm/μs	SHEAR (TRANSVERSE) WAVES IMPEDANCE Z_T = gm × 10³/cm²-s	SURFACE (RAYLEIGH) WAVES VELOCITY V_R = cm/μs	SURFACE (RAYLEIGH) WAVES IMPEDANCE Z_R = gm × 10³/cm²-s
AIR	0.001	0.033	0.33	-	-	-	-
ALUMINUM 1100-O	2.71	0.635	1,720	0.310	840	0.290	788
ALUMINUM, ALLOY 2117-T4	2.80	0.625	1,750	0.310	868	0.279	780
BARIUM TITANATE	0.56	0.550	310	-	-	-	-
BERYLLIUM	1.82	1.280	2,330	0.871	1,600	0.787	1,420
BRASS (NAVAL)	8.1	0.443	3,610	0.212	1,720	0.195	1,580
BRONZE (P-5%)	8.86	0.353	3,120	0.223	1,980	0.201	1,780
CAST IRON	7.7	0.450	2,960	0.240	1,850	0.193	1,720
COPPER	8.9	0.466	4,180	0.226	2,010	-	-
CORK	0.24	0.051	12	-	-	-	-
GLASS, PLATE	2.51	0.577	1,450	0.343	865	0.314	765
GLASS, PYREX	2.23	0.557	1,240	0.344	765	0.313	698
GLYCERINE	1.261	0.192	242	-	-	-	-
GOLD	19.3	0.324	6,260	0.120	2,320	-	-
ICE	1.00	0.398	400	0.199	199	-	-
LEAD, PURE	11.4	0.216	2,460	0.070	798	0.063	717
MAGNESIUM, ALLOY M1-A	1.76	0.574	1,010	0.310	539	0.287	499
MOLYBDENUM	10.09	0.629	6,350	0.335	3,650	0.311	339
NICKEL	8.8	0.563	4,950	0.296	2,610	0.264	2,320
OIL, TRANSFORMER	0.92	0.138	127	-	-	-	-
PLASTIC (ACRYLIC RESIN-PLEXIGLASS)	1.18	0.267	315	0.112	132	-	-
POLYETHYLENE	-	0.153	1,300	-	-	-	-
QUARTZ, FUSED	2.20	0.593	1,300	0.375	825	0.339	745
SILVER	10.5	0.360	3,800	0.159	1,670	-	-
STEEL	7.8	0.585	4,560	0.323	2,530	0.279	2,180
STAINLESS 302	8.03	0.566	4,550	0.312	2,500	-	-
STAINLESS 410	7.67	0.739	5,670	0.299	2,290	-	-
TIN	7.3	0.332	2,420	0.167	1,235	-	-
TITANIUM (Ti 150A)	4.54	0.610	2,770	0.312	1,420	0.279	1,420
TUNGSTEN	19.25	0.518	9,980	0.287	5,520	0.265	5,100
WATER	1.00	0.149	149	-	-	-	-
ZINC	7.1	0.417	2,960	0.241	1,710	-	-

NOTES